CW00621058

Men with Sexual Problems
and
What Women Can Do
to Help Them

Men with Sexual Problems
and
What Women Can Do
to Help Them

Eva Margolies, M.A., C.S.T.

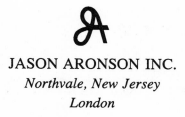

JASON ARONSON INC.
Northvale, New Jersey
London

This book was set in 11 pt. Times Roman by Alabama Book Composition of Deatsville, AL, and printed and bound by Book-mart Press, Inc. of North Bergen, NJ.

Library of Congress Cataloging-in-Publication Data

Margolies, Eva.
    Men with sexual problems and what women can do to help them / by Eva Margolies.
      p. cm.
    Previously published as: Undressing the American male. New York : Dutton, c1994.
    Includes index.
    ISBN 0–7657–0317–3
      1. Psychosexual disorders. 2. Men—Sexual behavior. 3. Sexual disorders.
    4. Sex therapy. I. Margolies, Eva. Undressing the American male. II. Title.

  RC556 .M36 2001
  616.85'83'0081 — dc21

                                    00–067545

Printed in the United States of America on acid-free paper. For information and catalog write to Jason Aronson Inc., 230 Livingston Street, Northvale, NJ 07647-1726, or visit our website: www.aronson.com

To the men who had the courage
to open their hearts to me

Contents

PART TWO
WHAT YOU CAN DO

Preface

This is a book for women who want to know about men's sexual problems and how to deal with them.

I am writing it because despite the many volumes written on sexuality, not one is specifically directed toward helping women deal with men who have sexual problems.

I am writing it because over the course of more than twenty years as a sex therapist, I have come to empathize with the profound effect that having a sexual problem has on a man's sense of self-worth.

I am writing it because the men who have so generously and trustfully confided their innermost secrets and fears have given me a new perspective and a new respect for how fragile the male psyche can be.

I am writing it because often, without realizing it, women significantly contribute to, perpetuate, and in some cases actually trigger many of the sexual problems men experience, but they can also be the pivotal force in helping men resolve them.

What are the chances that you or a woman you know will encounter a man with a sexual problem? Although there are no definitive statistics, there is every reason to believe that the woman who has *not* encountered such a man is the exception. Recent studies estimate that about 30 percent of all men suffer from premature ejaculation and another 10 percent suffer from erectile dysfunctions,* the new euphemism for impotence. These statistics do not include men who suffer from too little or too much sexual desire or paraphilia or fetishes. Nor do the statistics include gender-confusion disorders and sexual shyness and inhibition.

When we take all these problems into account, it is not a far leap to believe that if about 40 percent of all males suffer from a sexual problem, then the majority of females have been with such a man. Even so, I have been amazed by the lack of understanding most women have about male sexuality and sexual functioning. What comes across to a man at best as inconsideration, and at most as blatant contempt, from a woman is more often than not her sheer ignorance.

Most women do not know, for example, that men with premature ejaculation are not sexually selfish but are completely unable to control their orgasms. Nor are most women aware that erection problems, particularly at the beginning of a new relationship, are almost never a sign of a man's lack of attraction for his partner. And the majority of women are completely oblivious of the thousands of thirty-, forty-, and even fifty-year-old men who suffer from sexual shyness and inexperience. Indeed, the high-powered, single CEO who constantly rejects the advances of women is possibly suffering from some sort of sexual problem or feelings of inadequacy.

Obviously, we cannot respond appropriately to what we do not understand. The result is a great male–female sexual chasm in which men feel unheard and inadequate and women feel rejected or used. It is the purpose of this book to fill that gap, to give women an understanding of the complexity of male sexual problems as well as to provide them with the tools that can help resolve them.

Contrary to what many writers on the subject would have you believe, male sexual problems are complex. In addition, the problems

---

*Bernie Zilbergeld, Ph.D., quoted in Shelley Levitt, "His Sexuality: Special Report," *New Woman* (November 1991), p. 100.

men experience often occur in combination. Knowing the themes and variations of each problem is important because for you to begin resolving the dysfunction, you first must understand what is causing it.

This book will also address the way that we, as women, sometimes contribute to, exacerbate, and even cause male sexual problems through our ignorance and sexual biases. You will be asked to look at your own sexuality and feelings about men in general and about men with sexual problems in particular.

In addition, this book is not only about men's sexual problems but about the men who have these problems. I will discuss how men's feelings about having a sexual problem affect their self-image as well as their feelings about women. I will talk about the personality of the man who has the problem and how this relates to the problem he is experiencing and his prognosis for overcoming it. Dealing with a premature ejaculator who is easygoing, as opposed to a premature ejaculator whose personality is rigid and controlling, makes for two very different stories.

In some ways this is a how-to book. You will be given up-to-date information about the male body and sexual functioning. For example, what medications affect male sexual response? Is there a certain type of penis structure that is associated with impotence? In the chapters on treatment, I will describe exercises and techniques that you can practice and that can successfully alleviate the problem. You will learn how to be a teacher, a kind of sexual coach. You will learn what you should look for as you practice the exercises and how you can tell if your partner is responding in a way that's helping him overcome the problem.

This is also a how-not-to book. Often, usually unintentionally, women say or do things that only exacerbate existing problems, so I will spend considerable time discussing the kinds of things you need to avoid.

Finally, this is a when-to, when-not-to as well as a whom-to, whom-not-to book. Knowing when and when not to help and whom and whom not to help can go a long way toward alleviating a woman's disappointment and frustration. Not all men with sexual problems are interested in being helped. Others may be very interested, but the kind of help they need may be far beyond what you can provide. Once you have read this book, you will know how to pinpoint the men who are worth the effort and to avoid those who will never be satisfying partners no matter how hard you try.

Acknowledgments

There are several people whom I would like to thank.

Jason Aronson was unwavering in his enthusiasm for this book.

I am also very grateful to my colleagues at Center for Sexual Recovery who shared their insights and expertise with me.

Finally the patients, whose identifying characteristics have been significantly altered to preserve their anonymity, have a special place in my heart. Their honesty and trust made this book possible.

PART ONE

MEN'S
SEXUAL
PROBLEMS

1

The Naked Truth

Richard, a pleasant-looking man, is thirty-nine and earns close to half a million dollars a year working for a major airline. He gives speeches worldwide and has a wry sense of humor that often earns him the reputation of the life of the party. Yet although he desperately wants to get married and to have children, he dates infrequently. That is because Richard is a virgin. During one of our sessions he becomes angry at me when I tell him I understand how bad he must feel about his situation. "You haven't the vaguest, foggiest idea of how I feel," he says accusingly.

"Women don't believe me." "Women don't understand." "Women can't imagine what it is like." These are the plaints of men whose self-esteem has been battered, whose self-respect has been destroyed. These are men who suffer not only from sexual problems but from the emotional scars those problems create. These are the men who need women to be there for them, to understand, but who fear they do not or cannot.

How many such men are there? Recent statistics suggest that close to *half of all men* experience a sexual problem at one time or another in their lives! Given this astounding fact, one would think that most women would be sensitive to this possibility instead of being shocked upon encountering such a man. But the sad truth is that all too often women are not sensitive. I have been shocked by the minuscule number of patients who have told me that their partners responded in a supportive way, saying, "I see there is a problem here. What do we need to do to resolve it?" On the contrary, the overwhelming number of women react in a manner that is ultimately detrimental. Some, for example, inappropriately blame themselves. Others pretend that it doesn't matter. This, of course, only perpetuates the problem. Others, particularly if they are fifty or older, act as if a partner's loss of functioning is a fait accompli, which is like signing a death warrant to one's sex life. And some women are outright hostile, fueling a common fantasy among men that when they do not perform well, their ineptitude will be the talk of the town. (One man told me that his wife, in a fit of anger, threatened to tell everyone they knew that he was a premature ejaculator.)

Even when a woman wants to be understanding, she often does not understand. That is because most women are extremely ignorant about healthy male sexual functioning and know even less about men's sexual problems. Most women, for example, do not know that men with premature ejaculation have absolutely no control over their climaxes, even though most desperately wish that they did. Many women experience frustration or, in some cases, outright anger at partners who ejaculate prematurely. The fact that a woman feels unsatisfied because she does not climax during intercourse as the result of her partner's lack of control is only part of what rattles her. Given her erroneous assumption that the premature ejaculator could last longer if he really wanted to, she takes his lack of control as an insult. Feeling used for his own selfish pleasure, she understandably begins responding negatively, and this only increases his anxiety. The result is that he comes even more quickly and often begins avoiding sex altogether.

Even less understood than premature ejaculation are the erectile dysfunctions. If you have ever been with a man who has lost it during sex, chances are your first response has been to feel rejected or inadequate. "What's wrong with me?" you probably asked yourself.

"Why don't I turn him on?" Yet in truth, only a small percentage of erection problems are the result of a man's lack of attraction to his partner. Erectile dysfunctions have a panoply of causes. In some cases a man who is capable of functioning may simply be suffering from a powerful performance anxiety that makes him a bundle of unresponsive nerves. This is particularly true when he is with a woman he likes and wants to please. Chronic erection problems, however, generally signal deeper troubles. These include low self-esteem, unconscious negative feelings about the man's present relationship, a history of emotional incest or sexual abuse, and a fear of or anger toward women that often goes back to his relationship with his mother. The performance anxiety these men experience is not your normal garden variety but a powerful childlike terror of being rejected or humiliated.

A woman's ignorance about male sexuality can also be a primary trigger in a chronic erection problem. Most women, and men, too, have bought into the mythology that a man should always be ready, willing, and able to have sex when there is an available woman in the vicinity. In addition, they may share the erroneous assumption that a man is supposed to get an erection without any kind of direct stimulation. I am not saying that men don't get spontaneous erections. However, as men age, the ability to "get it up" simply from the mental aspects of arousal diminishes in most of them. Not infrequently what you have are a man and a woman, both ignorant about normal sexual functioning, both operating under the assumption that erections are supposed to appear miraculously. When they don't, the man starts to panic, and his partner begins to wonder what's wrong with her. Perhaps she even becomes angry. Neither partner understands that it is perfectly natural and possibly necessary for her to stimulate his penis in order to produce an erection. The result is an increasing number of unsatisfying sexual encounters, which can eventually end in complete impotence.

Obviously the rarer the disorder, the less information women have about it. Lack of desire and what I call disorders of inexperience (yes, there are many more thirty- and forty-year-old virgins than you can imagine) so fly in the face of what we think of as adequate sexual functioning for men that few women have much tolerance for dealing with men who experience these problems. Even men who suffer from simple sexual shyness tend to be the target of female rejection and outright disdain, even though they often are functional and can enjoy sex a great deal. Ironically, with just a little bit of support and understanding, many of these men have the potential to be excellent lovers and husbands.

Finally, a woman's inhibitions about sex can have a profound effect on male sexual functioning and response. One patient came to me completely impotent after his wife of one-and-one-half years left him because he was "too kinky." Upon questioning, I learned that "too kinky" meant that he enjoyed having his balls stimulated by her fingers during lovemaking. Occasionally, too, he enjoyed experimenting by placing whipped cream or a liqueur on her body and licking it off. Both these activities were given such bad press by his wife he began to feel he was a pervert. Because he felt oppressed by her rejection, they had sex less and less frequently. Over time his interest in her, and in sex generally, subsided to the point of his being unable to get an erection even while masturbating.

The bottom line is that most women, through no fault of their own, are completely ignorant about men's sexual needs and male sexual functioning. Be honest. Like most women, you probably subscribe to the idea that men are supposed to be the sexual conquistadors. They are supposed to be the ones to initiate, especially at the beginning of a relationship. They are supposed to be our sexual mentors. We expect them to know how to be great lovers.

The more macho the culture, the grander the demands. To be a white American male and be less than stud of the year is one thing. To be Latino or African-American and have a sexual problem is, to many men and women, a contradiction in terms. One sexually inexperienced black male came to me in utter frustration after attempting to learn how to be a good lover from the women he was dating. "When I have asked women to tell me what they like, they have just laughed. 'Oh, you know what to do.' They just assume that because I'm black, I'm hung and a stud."

Sadly, men often don't live up to these lofty expectations. And most of us are in the dark when it comes to helping them.

Of course, women's ignorance is only part of the problem. It is indeed difficult to develop an understanding of men with sexual problems when men do psychological somersaults to hide the fact that they have problems or, when the problems are blatantly obvious, to mask their shame about them. The shame and stigma that are associated with having a sexual problem are so powerful that most men devise all sorts of mechanisms to avoid dealing directly with it. Some men frequent prostitutes as a way of covering up their feelings of inadequacy. A good call girl is attractive and compassionate. She knows how to flatter a man, and for a male whose modus operandi is to run away from his problem and affirm his masculinity, that flattery means everything.

Other men hide their problems behind what comes across as a controlling and sometimes noxious facade. Men who are hiding erection problems, for example, often appear forceful, brazen, charming, and at the same time terribly distrustful and angry in a controlled sort of way. When such a man shows up for treatment, what I usually see is someone who is well dressed, who sits with his legs crossed, his arms spread out on the top of the couch, who asks about my credentials with a paranoiac skepticism, and who engages in a real battle of wills when asked to commit to a program of treatment. If the problem is premature ejaculation or inhibited male orgasm, add to the disguise a look that is simultaneously leering and degrading. This is the man who looks you up and down in a derogatory, almost menacing kind of way and, if he is over forty-five, condescendingly calls you "dear." (Of course, there are always exceptions. I will never forget the little Jewish man who was seventy plus but swore he was "fifty-tree," who, after being reassured that his problem was solvable, told me in earnest appreciation that "you are a very sweet girl, darlink.")

Men's paranoia about being seen anywhere in the vicinity of a sex therapy clinic is another sign of their profound sense of embarrassment about having a sexual problem. Even though my office is in an institute with many other health practitioners, I have had many a patient tell me that he has actually gone to another floor if someone in the elevator, usually another male, looked at him cockeyed. This dynamic has provided a business boom to the hobby shop in the building, my patients' favorite escape hatch. Several patients have told me that they have seen acquaintances in the shop. Unbeknownst to any of them, all were patients of mine.

Not surprisingly, this paranoia about being discovered also translates into a strong aversion to sitting in the waiting room. Not infrequently, when I come out to get a patient, he is hiding behind a newspaper. Others pace the floor or remain in the bathroom until their appointed time. Still others refuse to wait at all. Indelibly etched in my mind is the picture of a handsome and imposing-looking man, impeccably dressed, sitting on the couch in my office reading *People* magazine. I had never met him before, and I was a few minutes late for our appointment. Refusing to sit in the waiting room for fear of being seen, this man walked right past the receptionist and into my private office. By the time I arrived, he looked quite at home. I found myself feeling very irritated by this audacious invasion, a feeling that turned into compassion when he said, staring me straight in the eye but suddenly looking small and timid, "I am about to tell you something I've never told anyone before. I have never been able to have successful intercourse with anyone but my ex-wife. I'm terrified that someone will find out that I'm impotent." Most women, meeting this man, would see someone physically, intellectually, and professionally arresting. It would be almost impossible to guess that behind his imposing veneer there was an extraordinarily fragile sense of masculinity. This man's feelings of inadequacy were so profound that they prevented him from continuing therapy. The emotional upheaval that would have been necessary to discover the taproots of his problem required his giving up more emotional control than he was able to muster. As much as he wanted help, he was unable to overcome the humiliation of having shared his darkest secret with me.

Even men who do enter treatment are intensely guarded when they first come in for therapy. I am still struck by how long it takes most men to be themselves with me and the great lengths to which they will go not to be found out. The stigma they attach to having sexual problems is so strong that it is not uncommon for a patient not to tell me his real name until he has known me for a while. Most eventually confess their true identities, of course, although I have had a couple of patients who completed treatment without telling me their real names.

Withholding one's name not only negatively affects the therapeutic relationship but in one instance almost led to a devastating encounter. About a year ago a handsome young man suffering from a serious erection problem came in for help. At the beginning of treatment he was not very forthcoming about his history and experiences growing up. He did not give me his real name. When pressed, though, he did tell me that his parents' relationship was a constant battlefield. He snidely attributed this to his mother's Irish temper and his father's Scandinavian passivity. At the same time I was also seeing another man in his fifties from Norway who was locked in a miserable marriage and was suffering extreme premature ejaculation. One evening the two had back-to-back appointments. At the last minute the older man canceled, saying he had an emergency at the restaurant he owned. Fifteen minutes after that call, the younger man called to tell me that he couldn't make his appointment because there was an emergency in his father's restaurant. It did not take long for me to realize that I was treating father and son, both of them using false names.

One of the most humorous and at the same time one of the saddest stories of how painful getting professional help for a sexual problem can be is of a young man who was referred to me by his family doctor. My first contact with Joe was over the phone. It was a call that one does not easily forget. "Hi. My name is Joe Baretta. I was referred to you by Dr. Matheus. I would like to set up an appointment with you, but I'm sort of nervous about it. Can you tell me what happens when I come in?"

"Well," I answered gently, "we just talk a little bit about the problem you have been experiencing, and then I will be able to tell you how we can go about solving it."

At this point a hand went over the receiver, and I heard Joe say, "Hey, it's no big deal. You just go in and talk to her, and she will tell you why your dick isn't working."

"It sounds as if you are really nervous about this," I responded, getting the gist of what was occurring. "Do you think it would help if we set up an appointment in the near future? I have some time on Thursday around three in the afternoon. You might feel more reassured after coming in."

"Good idea," he answered. Hand over the receiver again: "Can you get off work Thursday in the afternoon?" Then back to me: "Three o'clock is fine."

When Thursday came around, I was expecting to see a bunch of rattled nerves, to say the least. On the contrary, the patient seemed fairly collected. The only problem was that he was having difficulty answering some of the questions I was asking him.

"Okay," I said, "so you've been losing your erection when intercourse becomes imminent for about six months now. What happens when you masturbate?"

"Umm, well, I'm not exactly sure," came the response.

"Well, do you lose your erection during masturbation, or can you stimulate yourself to orgasm?"

More hesitation. "Well, the truth is I don't know because . . ."

It finally dawned on me. Joe was not actually Joe but his best friend. Too afraid and too ashamed to come in himself, he sent his friend on a reconnaissance mission to my office to make sure there were no land mines. Eventually Joe did come in to see me, and we were able to resolve his problem successfully. But getting him there was obviously no small task.

Once patients are committed to therapy, there is still the awkwardness almost all of them have about what language to use with me. Invariably most early sessions sound like something out of a high school textbook with everything we discuss having at least three syllables. There are plenty of problems with "ejaculation" and "sexual intercourse" and issues surrounding "manual stimulation" versus "fellatio." A lot of men, trying to explain their problems, will question me outright about what kinds of words they should use. I always tell them to use whatever words come to mind, a response that is often met with "But those are words that I use with guys, and you're a lady." On occasion even my own attempt to ease the situation by using the vernacular is met by an embarrassed response. One twenty-eight-year-old computer analyst who had a problem climaxing with intercourse, for instance, broke up laughing when I asked him if he was able to come with any other kind of stimulation. "I'm sorry," he said apologetically. "It's just that 'come' seems like such a blue word for a woman therapist."

Of course, there is the man who goes to the other extreme. In an attempt to hide his shame, he will try to shake my composure by sounding like something that just crawled out of the sewer. Cool and composed, he begins by telling me he "has a thing for big tits," how he "loves to fuck" and prefers "a blow job to a hand job." The problem is just that he has "this little problem with coming" before he wants to (which in cases like these usually means he comes in thirty seconds or less). And even though his lover isn't really unhappy, he is a man who is always trying to improve every aspect of himself.

Eventually we do develop a comfort zone. In fact, the flip side of all this uneasiness and paranoia is that once I earn a man's trust, there is very little he will not tell me. Like a dam that has suddenly broken, a floodgate of emotion about his insecurities comes tumbling out. First, and almost across the board, there is this onset of hypersensitivity to any remark, even a positive one, that remotely has to do with sexual performance. What at one time might have been a man's dream can be twisted into his worst nightmare after he starts having difficulty with his functioning.

"Now, you have to imagine this," said one thirty-three-year-old advertising executive who had been having erection problems. "This really gorgeous girl approaches me at a party at Southampton and asks me to take a walk with her on the beach. It is late at night, and the beach is pretty empty. We are having what seems to be a pleasant conversation when she turns around and looks me straight in the eyes." By now he is wringing his hands. "And she says, 'I want you to boff my brains out.' My God! It's a fantasy come true. And all I can think is 'Get me the hell out of here.'"

Another man in his mid-fifties had a similar tale of woe. He had regained his ability to have erections with masturbation after many years of impotence, and we had finally gotten to the point in treatment where he felt courageous enough to consider "trying out the equipment" with a partner. He was courting a woman who was obviously hot for him, and their lovemaking seemed imminent. That is, until the fatal remark. As they drove home after a lovely evening, an old Carly Simon song, "Nobody Does It Better," aired on the radio. "I'll bet that can be said of you," his lady friend said coyly. The pressure to perform that he felt in response to this off-the-cuff remark produced such intense anxiety that it was the last time he saw her.

Then, of course, there is the perennial insecurity about penis size. I have come to believe that condoms should come in two sizes only: large and extra-large. I would bet money that there is hardly an American male who has not, at least on one occasion, measured his penis with a ruler and tape measure to gauge how satisfactorily his appendage sizes up in both length and breadth. And unless he is hung larger than an elephant, chances are he wishes it were, well, just a teeny bit bigger. The exception is the rare man who considers himself "well hung" and who invariably has a surreptitious way of passing on this information to me early in treatment.

What is a typical semiobsession among sexually functional men can become a real sore spot in a man who is questioning his sexuality. Larry is a case in point. Feeling like "a sexual novice" after divorcing his sexually unresponsive wife of twenty years, Larry claimed that he had a slightly smaller-than-average-sized penis, "maybe five inches erect or five and a quarter if I am really hard, and kind of on the skinny side." After spending a number of sessions discussing how women enjoy being pleasured sexually and explaining, again, and again, that the size of a penis is not all that important, he finally got up the gumption to ask out a woman he knew from the health club whom he had his eye on. The woman readily accepted, and after a number of dates it was clear that she was interested in progressing past the good-night kiss stage. I thought Larry, feeling increasingly confident as a result of her attention, was off to the races.

It was not meant to be. After a Saturday night movie the pair were sitting in a coffee shop when the couple in the next booth were served a super-hero on a loaf of sourdough bread. "I think I will buy myself a dildo like that," said Larry's potential lover, referring to the bread. What was, in all likelihood, meant as a rather explicit come-on sent Larry running in the opposite direction. "All I could see was her look of terrible disappointment when she saw my little chicken neck of a penis." The next time they spoke on the phone, he told her he had met someone else and was no longer interested in seeing her.

While some men run away from what they perceive as the source of intimidation, others try all sorts of maneuvers to counter it. Seeking out situations in which they know they will not be rejected is an extremely common ploy. One middle-management corporate executive who had a chronic problem sustaining his erections with his wife was a frequent customer at local topless bars. He told me that he had become a kind of mentor to the younger dancers. "I tell them there are two golden rules of good dancing: Dance like you love what you're doing, and dance like there is no other guy in the world besides the one you're dancing for," he told me proudly. When I asked why he had adopted these rules and why he seemed so drawn to the topless bars, he seemed puzzled. "I do it because it's fun," he told me as if there could be no other reason. After a few months of therapy he began to see his behavior for what it really was. Going to the bars was a way of establishing a sense of masculinity he did not experience in the bedroom. And his role of mentor was a way of assuring that he would never be shown up at the go-go the way he was at home. "There is the unwritten competition at these places," he confided, "that is about whose tips get taken first. Not having your tip accepted early is like standing with your dick in your hand and someone telling you, 'It isn't good enough.' Since the girls know and respect me, they never put me in this embarrassing position."

The desire never to be shown up explains why so many men prefer going to massage parlors that offer a hand job for an additional fee to going to prostitutes. An engineer who felt inadequate because none of the women he had been with (including his wife) had ever had an orgasm explained it: "If I went to a prostitute, there would still be the issue of trying to satisfy her, and her probably faking it, and not knowing if you did or not. At the massage houses you are passive and don't have to worry about pleasing your partner. That takes a lot of the pressure out of it."

Still others create in fantasy what they cannot do in real life. "A recurrent theme in my sexual fantasies is that I am stud of the year," one fifty-year-old man told me. "Most of my fantasies begin with my walking into a large club of some sort where there are all these beautiful women. A few of the better-looking ones compete for my attention, and finally one wins out. She suggests we leave. The next scene is us on the bed and we are having intercourse. She is coming again and again and telling me I am the best lover she has ever had." In his imagination this man can last forever. In reality he has a long history of premature ejaculation that has recently been compounded by difficulty sustaining an erection.

As profound as the feelings of inadequacy is the staggering ignorance many of these man share about both the male and female sexual facts of life. I am constantly amazed by the lack of knowledge among men who are otherwise competent and sophisticated. When I first began working with men, I made the mistake of judging a man's education about sex by his social cover. If he was well-to-do, cultured, and married, I assumed he also knew his sexual ABC's, so I skipped over a lot of sex education stuff that I would discuss with patients I suspected were ignorant. That all changed when I was talking to a forty-three-year-old man who owned a chain of automotive stores and was married with three children. We were discussing about how he might try massaging his wife's clitoris during intercourse since the clitoris is the primary sex organ for the female. I remember the dumb-founded look on his face. "What's wrong?" I asked, unable to interpret why his jaw had suddenly dropped to his knees. "I always thought that a woman's main sex organ was her tits," he said with a combination of awe and embarrassment.

He, I quickly learned, was far from the only one. Although most men these days know of the clitoris, many admit they are not exactly sure, when touching a woman, if they have found the right spot. Believe it or not, I even treated a gynecologist who said that finding a woman's clitoris during lovemaking often defied him. Then there is the man who has found the right spot but has not figured out that a woman who purportedly can't come during intercourse could easily climax if her clitoris were stimulated during penetration.

Sadly, men are just as unknowledgeable about their own bodies and functioning. A great number of men haven't the foggiest idea where the prostate gland is or what it does. Others are not aware that a penis that is smaller when flaccid tends to increase proportionately more in size than an unaroused penis that is large—in essence, that a small and a large flaccid penis can be virtually identical after arousal. Still others do not know that it is perfectly natural for a penis to lose some of its rigidity as a man ages.

Then there are men who are factually knowledgeable in a general sense but have very little specific information about their partners. A striking number of men I have worked with are not certain if their partners are having orgasms. Even more have no idea about whether their significant others masturbate or simply can't fathom the idea. Almost always this is a direct result of their own embarrassment about asking the question and their fear of inadequacy about having the question answered. One man went for twenty years of married life assuming that his wife was unable to have orgasms because she never had one with him. When I pressed him to ask her about self-stimulation, he learned that she had orgasms regularly with masturbation. "I guess I never asked her about it because I didn't want to know the answer," he told me. "I mean, if she can have orgasms alone and not with me, what does that say about my ability as a lover?"

Even when they know the facts, men often can't believe them. I have done mental gymnastics trying to convince some men that penis size is not very significant to women. Even more exhausting is getting a man to accept that it is perfectly normal after a certain age to need direct stimulation in order to get and sustain an erection. In fact, some men need direct physical contact for arousal at a fairly young age. A lot of married men also have trouble dealing with the fact that most married men masturbate, that having a regular sexual partner, even a good sexual partner, does not replace what some men still view as "second-rate sex."

Then there is the seemingly unfathomable idea that other men— many other men, in fact—have sexual problems. Men do not talk to each other honestly about sex, so virtually every man that I work with is convinced that he is one of an inept minority. The secrecy surrounding having a sexual problem was underscored by a patient who referred a close friend of his to me for therapy. Friend A, let's call him John, was a suave, sophisticated, seemingly has-it-all-together male in his mid-thirties who had one of the worst cases of premature ejaculation I had ever treated. Although outwardly he projected confidence, inwardly he was extremely anxious and insecure. His embarrassment about the problem not only made the problem worse but led him to go from woman to woman, only to retreat in shame once the relationship became sexual.

As John was beginning to overcome his problem, he referred his friend Daniel to me. He did not tell Daniel that he was seeing me himself but rather said that his internist had recommended me. You can imagine how shocked I was when David held John out as the epitome of virility. "This guy has an absolutely incredible way with women," he told me. "I've never seen someone so adept at getting women to go to bed with him." When I suggested that all is not always what it seems, that perhaps John had his own insecurities, Daniel quickly disputed the idea. "Absolutely not," he told me. "John brags about his prowess, about how he can last and make women come again and again. If only I could be like him!" If this is what close friends tell each other, one can imagine the distortions that are flung between locker room buddies.

The most difficult thing of all for a man with sexual problems to believe, however, is that any woman, even one he is in a long-term relationship with, can respect a man with any sort of sexual problem. It does not matter how good-looking or how much money he makes. A man with a sexual problem believes that he is seriously defective as a male, and he projects those feelings onto everyone around him.

This powerful fear of being unacceptable to a woman is, I think, why a man's strong desire to share, to open up, and to be known is not infrequently counterbalanced by an equally strong desire to come across as having it all together, as "masculine." There is this push-pull, this approach-avoidance to being vulnerable that men share. Sometimes this comes across as a sudden coldness. One sexually inexperienced man in his early thirties, for instance, had an anxiety attack in my office and nearly fainted. When in the next session we discussed what had occurred, he told me that he had been furious with me for having given him a masturbation assignment. "Maybe I don't know much about women, but I have plenty of experience doing it on my own, thank you," he said snidely. In the mire of the anger we got to the hurt: the feeling of intimidation about talking to a woman about being a virgin, the sensitivity to rejection, and the terror of such rejection. For a few moments this man, who was difficult to feel a connection to because he intellectualized everything, was very real, very close. He felt it, too, because almost without warning, he sat up straight and said, "I thought this was sex therapy. Do I have to bare my soul to overcome my virginity?"

"Probably not," I responded honestly.

"That's good," he said, getting up and almost slamming the door behind him.

While usually not this dramatic, the desire to shut down after opening up is very common. When I first began working intensely with men, I remember wondering why, after treatment was over, they rarely called or wrote to let me know how they were doing. When following up on their progress myself, I learned that even though they very much appreciated the help I had given them, and for many, I held a special place in their hearts, I and everything associated with me—their problems specifically—were a part of their lives that they wanted to forget, to pretend had never happened.

Although the trials men go through to hide their problems may sound extreme, keep in mind that these men, having sought help, are the more open ones. Vulnerability and dependency are traits that women accept in themselves. Most men, on the other hand, have great difficulty admitting they have a problem and an even harder time going for therapy to resolve it. For every man I see, there are a hundred more who suffer silently and alone. These are the men who avoid women completely. The fear of humiliation and failure is so overpowering that they would rather give up their sex lives than lose what they perceive as their masculinity and self-respect.

If the fact that men with sexual problems are in hiding is a great deal of the problem, then helping men come out of hiding is a great deal of the solution. In many ways that is what this book is all about. Having helped hundreds of patients over the years, I have gained appreciation and empathy for the suffering that men with sexual problems experience. I have learned what these men need, how they think, and how to help them. I have come to have a profound respect for how much courage it takes, how brave a man must be to confess, "I have a sexual problem." I feel privileged because I have seen so many men go through a sexual and emotional metamorphosis. When a man undresses, when he exposes his vulnerability, he develops a tremendous capacity for what women crave but so often fail to get from men: true intimacy. Here I will pass on this privileged information and, in the process, teach you to help a man resolve his problem.

2

Men Who
Come Too Fast

Hal is a fifty-year-old insurance salesman who makes more than half a million dollars a year. He took his street smarts, which he acquired growing up in a rough neighborhood on the outskirts of Los Angeles, and applied them to the world of high finance. He makes his living by talking fast. He owns three state-of-the-art sports cars, and he drives fast. And he has a wife who is on the brink of divorcing him because he comes fast.

He is not atypical of a certain type of premature ejaculator, and I am having a hard time feeling much sympathy for him. He is talking so loudly that I know that everyone on the floor is going to be a privy to the intimate details of his sex life. I find myself, despite my best efforts to do otherwise, psychologically siding with his wife, who is not there because she has reached the point of giving up. I am not sure I blame her. If his lovemaking is anything near as irritating as his initial presentation—and I have every reason to believe that it is, as he tells me in a rat-a-tat-tat staccato how "first I play with her tits and then I guess I move down to her clit and then I rub it for a while until she comes because I know I can't hold off and then I put it in and come and she gets mad because she isn't getting enough"—his wife deserves all the sympathy in the world.

Then, out of the clear blue, I see tears forming in his eyes. "I want to be a better lover so that my wife will stay with me. She thinks I don't care, but that isn't true. I just don't know how to do what she wants. I worked myself up from the ghetto. I earn more in one year than my father made in his lifetime. But being able to hold back when I am having sex absolutely defies me."

He is far from alone. Premature ejaculation (PE) is extremely common, so much so, in fact, that it is estimated that about one-third of the adult male population suffers from it. That's many millions of men. And while not as crushing as erection problems, PE has some nasty psychological effects on the men who experience it.

Not being able to control when a man comes can have a terrible effect on a marriage like Hal's. Being a premature ejaculator also puts a serious damper on most men's confidence not only as lovers but as men. Luke is a perfect example. At twenty-eight he is a hunk by anyone's definition. Six two, broad-shouldered, and with a smile that jumps out at you from his well-crafted face, he is the type of man that has heads turning on the street. But Luke rarely risks having a sexual encounter with a woman because of what he calls his sexual inadequacy. "Women have this image of me," he says straightforwardly and without arrogance. "I know I am handsome, and women expect me to follow through by being a great lover. But once I get into a sexual encounter, that image is totally blown away by this premature thing. It has been so humiliating that I now break off relationships right at the point when things look as if they are going to become sexual."

I try to reassure Luke that his problem is resolvable, that many men suffer from it, and that it has nothing to do with how masculine he is—all to no avail. "Look," he says, leaning toward me and looking straight into my eyes, "I know you're trying to help me. But frankly I don't give a flying you-know-what if the whole world has this problem. Let's face it, popping off like a jackrabbit isn't exactly what you would call studly."

A man who is otherwise suave, successful, and socially gregarious but who comes quickly often tells me he feels he is living his life as an impostor. "I only look together," said Evan, who is twenty-four, charming, and enormously wealthy. "But as soon as I get into the bedroom, it's all over. They know the *real* me." Unlike Luke, who opted to cut off his sex life, Evan developed a different tactic to deal with the humiliation of not living up to what he believed was the proper image: He became a bed hopper. "I never go to bed with someone more than once or with anyone who might have any chance of knowing anyone I know. That way I never really have to be found out." When I asked Evan how he intended ever to get into a long-term relationship, he was at a loss. And when I first suggested to him that he simply tell a potential sexual partner that he has a problem, he looked at me as if I were a Martian. (I make this suggestion because even though a man might find it initially embarrassing, it is less embarrassing than having the problem without any forewarning. Also, confiding in a partner about the possibility of having a problem often helps reduce a man's anxiety about performing, which can have the positive effect of improving his functioning.)

If having the problem can wreck the self-esteem of the man who is otherwise socially adept, it can totally devastate the man who is shy to begin with and can eventually turn him into a social hermit. One absolutely adorable Latino in his late twenties had been so traumatized by his quick-on-the-trigger performance that he had not been out on a date for six years. "It took me six months to get up the gumption to ask out this girl Monica that I had a crush on," he confessed shyly. "It took me another six months to get up the nerve to sleep with her. But it only took me six seconds to come." He shook his head. "So," he asked, "is it going to take me six years to solve this problem?"

Of course, not all premature ejaculators follow the road down the great retreat from intimacy. Many men with this problem try to ignore it or get around it by becoming great lovers in ways that don't involve their penises. But the humiliation and embarrassment, though often less obvious, persist. "I always make sure to give my wife an orgasm before I come," one man told me, because afterward I feel so ashamed that I can't look at her."

The shame is often transformed into outright terror when a man's partner brings the problem into the open. Even if their partners are understanding, many men begin harboring the fear that their lovers will find men with greater staying power if the problem is not resolved. And if a man's partner is not particularly sympathetic—and as I shall discuss shortly, many are not—he can become so distraught that his anxiety makes him come even more quickly. In some cases he may even begin having difficulties with his erections. Sex, which is supposed to be a source of pleasure, becomes a dreaded event to be increasingly avoided.

Up until now I haven't even mentioned the effect that PE can have on a man's own sexual pleasure, and for good reason. It's obvious that coming too quickly makes it impossible to enjoy that slow, languorous buildup of sexual arousal, just as gulping down your food isn't as pleasurable as savoring each bite. But when men come in for treatment, their own pleasure is usually the last thing on their minds. In part this is because a number of premature ejaculators don't believe that they are missing out on anything. For them, orgasm is the thing, and as long as they come, they think that they *are* enjoying sex. Even among men who know that they are not really enjoying sex because they come too rapidly or because their desperate attempt to hold back takes the fun out of sex, their lack of physical pleasure pales in contrast with their feelings of inadequacy or their fears that they are not pleasing their partners. When, at the end of an intake interview, I ask men to tell me, in their own words, what they would most like to get from therapy, their responses are invariably performance-oriented:

- "I would like to be able to satisfy a woman the real way with my penis."
- "I want to last longer so women will think of me as a good lover."
- "I want to feel adequate as a man."
- "I want to develop control so my wife won't feel so frustrated and get so mad at me."

In fact, in all my years as a sex therapist only rarely has a man told me that his primary reason for overcoming premature ejaculation is so that he can have more sexual pleasure. And among the few men who do talk about wanting to enjoy sex more, that desire is usually an afterthought, something like "I'd like to give my partner more pleasure and feel good about myself as a lover . . . oh, and I guess it would be nice to last longer because I could enjoy sex more, too."

In reality, men with premature ejaculation are no more or less selfish than men who do not have premature ejaculation, although most women, as we shall discuss shortly, have a hard time believing this is so.

WHAT CONSTITUTES
A PREMATURE EJACULATOR?

Since just about every man ejaculates rapidly at one time or another, how can you tell if the man in your life actually has premature ejaculation?

The answer is not cut-and-dry. Over the years the definition of "premature ejaculation" has undergone considerable change.

A race against the clock: The earliest definitions of PE had men competing with the clock. A man had PE if he couldn't last a specified period of time after penetration, with some professionals putting the number at two minutes and others at ten or fifteen minutes. This definition quickly ran into problems because it did not take into account the fact that different women are slower or faster to have orgasm. What if a man could last ten minutes but it took his partner fifteen minutes?

A race against one's partner: Because professionals recognized the need to take a woman into account, the definition of PE was modified, with Masters and Johnson defining a premature ejaculator as someone who could not satisfy his partner with intercourse more than 50 percent of the time. (Why they thought 50 percent of the time was sufficient, I'll never understand.) This definition, however, put men in a race not against the clock, but with their partners. Talk about performance pressure!

Another problem this definition does not take into account is that more than two out of three normally functioning women have difficulty reaching orgasm solely through the thrusting of the penis in the vagina (although many can come with intercourse as long as there is additional clitoral stimulation occurring simultaneously). What this means is that many women would have trouble having an orgasm with vaginal thrusting even if a man could last forever!

The concept of ejaculatory control: Most recently a premature ejaculator has been defined as someone who is unable to have reasonable control over when he ejaculates. In other words, a man is considered to have premature ejaculation if he cannot voluntarily and fairly easily choose to remain at a pretty high pitch of arousal for a period of time, if he cannot, within reason, decide when he is going to come.

For the most part I like this last definition, although even here, the issue of performance cannot be avoided. As one of my patients pointed out to me, the onus to develop control still rests with the male. "After all," he said, "sex therapists could deal with premature ejaculation by teaching women to hurry up."

"You're right," I admitted. "After all, you don't call a woman who can come within twenty seconds after penetration a premature comer."

"No," he said with a classic PE twinkle of his eye. "You just call her."

THE PROBLEM WOMEN HATE

However you define it, premature ejaculation is not a problem women take to kindly.

Given how common premature ejaculation is, one might think that women would have some understanding, if not tolerance, for this problem. Not so! Unlike other disorders such as erection problems, which often arouse some compassion, PE triggers rancor and contempt from all too many women.

The most logical reason for the disgruntlement is that PE interferes with a woman's sexual pleasure. "It's like pleasure interruptus" is the way one wife described it. "I really enjoy intercourse, and just as

I'm starting to get into it, he either stops or comes." Also, since a lot of men with this problem avoid being on top because they experience more penile sensation in this position, the woman who loves the missionary position is out of luck.

If you're a woman who is orgasmic with penetration, the complaint is understandable. A man's inability to hold out can definitely be frustrating and downright upsetting, particularly if the only way you can come is with intravaginal containment. Yet while the complaint that PE makes intercourse less pleasurable is certainly legitimate, I have noticed that many women who have no tolerance for PE have great difficulty or are even unable to reach orgasm with penetration. Nor does the fact that many men make up for their less than cooperative penises with more than cooperative hands and mouths often make much of a difference. And some of the men whose partners are the most hostile are women who have difficulty having orgasms at all.

Why, then, all the contempt on the part of women? In part, it may be due to the fact that a sizable percentage of men who have PE frequently have less than endearing sexual styles. Hal is an exaggerated but accurate example of the tendency among men who have this problem to make love in a way that is harried and hurried. There is also another type of man with premature ejaculation who becomes extremely nervous around women and exhibits a kind of sexual timidity that is anything but attractive. Finally there is the type of man with premature ejaculation whose fear of inadequacy runs so deep that he develops a counterphobic response to the problem. Rather than appear sexually nervous or inept, he can become outright lewd. To say that he objectifies women is an understatement. With a man like this, even knowing that he has a problem and is greatly ashamed of it doesn't necessarily make you care a whole lot about him.

But there are also a great many men who come too fast and do not fall into any of these categories. These are normal, sensual men who are sexually adept except for the fact that they can't control their ejaculations. Yet women seem to have almost as negative a response to these men as to their less able counterparts.

What is this lack of sympathy about? It seems to me that it is not PE per se but what we interpret as the causes of premature ejaculation that really rattles us. Some women view a man's inability to have control as a sign of wimpiness and immaturity. "Kenny just can't hold out as long as other men I've been with," complained a twenty-six-year-old woman who had never had an orgasm with or without a partner. "This sounds terrible, but it makes me feel he is not really masculine."

More commonly, though, a woman's negative response is a direct offshoot of the long-standing view that a man with PE is sexually selfish and out for his own interests. This, of course, means that women are simply the vessels for men's pleasure, sex objects in the most degrading sense.

Unfortunately there are some men just like this, men who grope, come, and roll over, never bothering themselves with the task of giving their partners pleasure. But most men with PE, while they can be anxious, sexually immature, and clumsy, are not innately selfish and do try and want to satisfy their partners. Contrary to the myth, premature ejaculators have absolutely no control over their ejaculations, although they desperately wish they had.

Fortunately most, with proper training, can.

HOW SERIOUS IS PE?

It always irks me when therapists talk about "simple" PE as if it were an uncomplicated problem with a surefire solution. It is true that premature ejaculation is easier to spot and understand than other problems, like lack of desire. Most men who have the problem do not suddenly develop it but have always had it to one extent or another. So if you have been with him two or three times and he swears up and down that this has never happened to him before, I would tend not to believe him. (There can be the very slim possibility that he is so enamored of you, and so desperately wants to make a good impression, that his anxiety is causing the problem.) Resolving PE also can be less complicated than overturning other sexual problems because it is rarely, although I won't say never, rooted in a deeply buried psychological problem that first needs to be uncovered.

At the same time there are many variables that make a particular man's problem more or less easy to resolve. Far from a "simple" dysfunction, premature ejaculation is caused and exacerbated by a host of factors.

EXCESSIVE SEXUALIZED AROUSAL: PE'S NUMBER ONE CAUSE

By far the most common cause of PE is an exaggerated mental response to anything remotely sexual.

Every woman has come across the type of man who looks at her in a not really lascivious but ogling kind of way. He is the man who seems to have sex not only on the brain but just about everywhere else. He is what I call an excessive sexualizer; virtually every look and touch that relate to a woman are given a sexual connotation.

If you are astute, you can learn to detect men who are likely to have PE from a few basic cues:

- *His handshake feels like a caress.* If he rubs your hand in that hey-baby-nice-to-meet-you way, you can almost be assured that he will not last long in bed.
- *A friendly hug does not feel like a friendly hug.* If he is incapable of a great bear hug and can only hug and stroke at the same time, PE is likely to be lurking in his history.
- *When he looks you up and down, you don't think that he is undressing you with his eyes but that he is ogling you with the look of a lecherous adolescent.* While some very sexy men have a way of looking at a woman that is downright seductive, the sexualizer's look seems annoying and immature.

In a nutshell, the sexualizer is in such a state of anxious anticipation when it comes to sex that he seems to leapfrog his way to early orgasm. Here is how his mind works. Let's say you are on a date and are enjoying a fabulous dinner. In his mind, you are half naked and he is already getting turned on. By the time he takes you back to his apartment and you are actually getting undressed, his mind is on intercourse. And by the time you get through foreplay and actually get to intercourse, it's all over because mentally he's been having intercourse for the past half hour.

Not surprisingly, men who tend to be analyzers and to think ahead about most things are particularly prone to becoming excessive sexualizers and developing PE. So are men who tend to rush everything they do.

Some people (men especially) think that a man like this is oversexed. But the truth is, rarely is such a man truly sexy. How could he be, when he never remains in the moment long enough to enjoy what is going on?

Many of my patients who are profuse sexualizers claim they love sex when they start therapy, but what they really love is that brief, delicious moment called orgasm. All their sexual energy is focused on that goal, and little else matters or feels particularly good. The excessive sexualizer experiences physical sensation in one of two ways. It is sexual—and that to a sexualizer translates as feelings that lead directly to orgasm—or it is not pleasurable because it "doesn't feel like anything."

Not surprisingly excessive sexualizers are completely out of touch with their bodies. To them sex is first and foremost a mental experience, and the focus on the physical, except for orgasm, is secondary. A sizable number of men with PE are so physically disconnected that when I have them masterbate without using any sort of fantasy, they often find themselves struggling to get an erection, let alone have an orgasm. This lack of physical sensitivity, naturally, greatly contributes to a premature response. When a man does not know what is going on in his body and cannot readily identify varying levels of sensation, he is in no position to control what's happening and cannot delay his response.

One of the most frustrating things about dealing with many men who are excessive sexualizers is that they are convinced that the extent of their mental arousal is perfectly normal and desirable. They assume, in fact, that just about every man thinks as they do and believe that any man who does not isn't really interested in sex. But the kind of sexualized arousal that is a staple among many men who have premature ejaculation *is* different from the normal pattern of arousal in many ways:

- *Almost no touch is nonsexual.* A man with a more normal pattern of arousal is able to enjoy the pleasurable sensations of a hand, back, or even body massage from a woman without becoming aroused. The man with an overdose of sexualized arousal gets turned on from the most benign touch coming from a woman he's at all attracted to.
- *He tends to get more aroused when giving than when receiving.* Most men with good sexual functioning experience some level of arousal when giving their partners sexual pleasure. I call this phenomenon "pleasure through osmosis," that is, mentally taking in his partner's arousal as if it is his own. A man who sexualizes excessively and who is prone to PE, however, gets extremely aroused not only by giving his partner pleasure but by simply touching her. The extent of his mental arousal is so pervasive that he often gets as, and sometimes even more, turned on from giving than receiving—a surefire sign that he's out of touch with his body.
- *He lacks sensuality and moves too fast.* Although some sexualizers learn, out of social courtesy, to slow down, the natural inclination of the sexualizer is to touch in a rushed, insensitive way. In fact, a man of this type is often a downright sloppy toucher. Very rarely does he spend much time on sensual touching. He does not know how to enjoy a slow, languorous buildup to arousal.
- *He is unable to stay in the pleasure of the moment.* The sexualizer is always at least one step ahead, anticipating what is going to come next. As a result, he never really enjoys what is happening right now.
- *Even his fantasies tend to be unsensual and hurried.* With the exception of the immature man with PE whom I shall discuss shortly, the sexual fantasies of the sexualizer are much like the way he makes love. Among such men, foreplay is almost unheard of, and when it does exist, it is cursory. There is no

seduction, no buildup. On the contrary, when I ask such a man to describe the movie in his head when he masturbates, he is likely to tell me, "I am having intercourse," or "A woman is giving me oral sex." When I query whether this is where the fantasy actually begins, the answer invariably is yes. Naturally it is also where it ends.

In addition to these characteristics, there is a certain type of sexually immature, almost adolescent man whose sexualizing manifests itself in the following way:

- *He gets almost as aroused from kissing (which he tends to refer to as making out) as from genital contact.* Stuck at an adolescent stage of sexual development, these men get highly aroused from kissing and hugging. Interestingly they may become even more turned on from these activities than from genital stimulation, which they experience some discomfort with.

This immature type of premature ejaculation also tends to have a few other traits that make his callowness apparent:

- *He uses baby words to refer to sexual parts of the body and often asks, in a childlike tone of voice, for permission to touch them.* Whether he is twenty-four or seventy, you can spot the sexually regressed man when he begins talking about sex in the whiny voice of a five-year-old. Questions like "May I play with your boobies?" or "Could you touch my you-know-what?" are immature not only in content but also in tone and are an instant turnoff to a woman who is the least bit sexual.

  Often there is a disapproving mother in the history of a man like this. Ever fearful of being punished or rebuffed, he approaches sex from the vantage point of a wanting but fearful child. This anxiety around criticism can make his premature ejaculation problem pretty difficult to overcome. Worse yet, his self-image is diminished when a woman rejects him because of his infantile ways.

- *He may masturbate by rubbing against a pillow or mattress instead of using his hand.* While not always the case, a lot of sexually immature men stimulate themselves by humping against something. Psychologically this is a regressed form of self-stimulation because he is not actually touching himself— that is, he is not taking his penis in his hand and saying, "I am doing this for my own pleasure." More important, masturbating in this way tends to make it more difficult to develop ejaculatory control because the sensations are more diffused and less precise. As a result, it is harder for him to tell when he is getting close to climax, and this in turn makes it hard for him to make the appropriate adjustments to slow down at that point.

Whether a man has PE and is also sexually immature or only has PE, being on the receiving end of all this hurried lovemaking style is obviously not much fun. That is why so many women describe men with premature ejaculation as lousy lovers. It is not simply the PE that is the problem but the whole lovemaking style. The bottom line is that while men like this are usually not intrinsically selfish, they tend to be sexually unsophisticated and sometimes immature—characteristics that are readily amenable to change with proper training and guidance.

Sexualized Arousal and Intercourse, "The Biggie"

At this point you might be telling yourself: "The man I'm with is different. I guess he rushes a little, and it's true that he gets more turned on from touching me than maybe he should, but overall he's a pretty good and focused lover except when it comes to intercourse. That's when he loses it completely." There are quite a few men who fall into this category. While almost every man who suffers from premature ejaculation tends to sexualize, there are many men for whom heavy-duty sexualizing occurs around specific activities, either oral sex or, more often, intercourse. These are men who give intercourse a lot more sexual value than all other sexual activities.

In some cases intercourse is emotionally loaded, an activity burdened with guilt and anxiety. More often, however, this specific type of sexualizing is a throwback to adolescence, when intercourse was considered a "homerun," as well as to the message most of us received suggesting that sex *means* intercourse. If intercourse, then, is what real sex is all about, mentally intercourse is also much more arousing than any other sexual activity. The result is that on some level such a head gets to intercourse and thinks, albeit often subconsciously, something like this: "Wow! I'm really doing it!" This sends his arousal skyrocketing and causes him to lose touch with what he is feeling in his body at that moment and hence to come too quickly—sometimes almost immediately. Interestingly, in the sexual fantasies of men who sexualize around the act of intercourse, they frequently come at the moment of penetration as well.

Often these men experience a great deal of frustration about their problem because they simply cannot understand why their control is so good until intercourse is imminent. "My girlfriend can stimulate me manually forever without my feeling that close to orgasm," one man, whose experience is not atypical, told me. "But as soon as we get to penetration and especially when we start moving, I get so excited that I can't hold back much." Unable to explain their lack of control to themselves, these men tend to rationalize their less than adequate control in one of two ways. The first of these explanations is that intercourse simply feels so much better on a physical level than anything else. The other is that intercourse comes after a buildup of arousal during foreplay, so it must be perfectly normal to get extremely excited. Of course, neither of these arguments holds much weight. If you could measure the physical arousal that occurs with penetration, particularly before the pace becomes fast and furious, you would find that it is not intrinsically more arousing than other forms of stimulation. (Actually researchers have found that the most powerful orgasms are triggered by masturbation.) The notion that intercourse is arousing as the result of all this foreplay also loses credibility because when you tell a man who comes quickly with penetration to experiment by skipping the foreplay and going for intercourse almost right away, he still comes very quickly.

The truth is that most men who sexualize around intercourse usually put intercourse on a kind of pedestal. It is considered much more forbidden and erotic. The good news is that once a man comes to understand the source of his problems, he can be desensitized to his excessive arousal at the point of intercourse fairly easily.

Small Penises, Sexualized Arousal, and PE

There is a kind of sexualizing that occurs among a number of men that has more to do with body image concerns than with sex. As much as we may think that men are less vain about their physical appearance than women, men are absolutely obsessed about the sizes of their penises. (If you don't believe me, ask every man you know if he has ever measured his penis, with and without an erection. I will bet you cannot find one who has not.) This concern with penis size is a major contributor to the development of PE for some men.

Over the years I began to notice a correlation between men who described their flaccid penises as smaller than average and PE. For a long time this was an enigma to me until one young man put the pieces together. Having been active in sports in college, he could not help noticing that other men's flaccid penises were much larger. Nor did his first attempt at intercourse help. Nervous as a schoolboy, he did not have an immediate erection when he was undressed, at which point his lady of the hour pronounced, "Gee, for someone so well built, I'm surprised it's so small!"

The combination of these experiences led him to swear to himself that never again would a woman see him unless he was hard. After all, he had already ascertained that his erect penis was a perfectly normal six inches long. Thus, when he started kissing a woman and found he did not have a firm erection, he began to fantasize. God forbid they should reach the point when he would be in his underwear or, worse yet, buck naked, with just his small penis to show for it. This led to an increasing amount of sexualized arousal and the inevitable development of a PE problem.

The key here is to help men concerned with penis size to feel more comfortable with their bodies so that they do not develop the tendency to oversexualize their arousal and develop PE. Unfortunately, once premature ejaculation becomes a problem, the tendency to sexualize is fairly automatic and takes some time to reverse. In cases like this there is little doubt that prevention is the best medicine.

Sexualized Arousal and Erection Problems

Finally, some men oversexualize their arousal in hope of avoiding an erection problem. Usually these are men who have had difficulty maintaining erections in the past or who fear they might have some difficulty in the future. Often, but not always, they are men of a certain age who no longer get rock-hard spontaneous erections at the drop of a hat and who do not understand that it is perfectly normal to need direct physical stimulation. Their sexualizing is a kind of panic-driven way of trying to arouse themselves. The result is that instead of having to deal just with their erection problem, they now have to deal with premature ejaculation as well.

Although we will discuss men with both premature ejaculation and erection problems in detail in the following chapter, it is important to say here that helping these men overcome their premature ejaculation is often extremely difficult until they resolve their erection problem. If a man has both dysfunctions, there is no doubt that resolving the erection problem is the number one priority. When a man who is afraid he has lost his masculinity because he is having trouble with his erections is told to just to focus on what he is feeling in his body, even if those sensations do not produce an erection, that is an awesome psychological task for him, one that meets great resistance. The result is a catch-22 in which the man mentally arouses himself to get an erection but comes too quickly because of all that mental arousal.

ANXIETY: PE'S NUMBER TWO CAUSE

Although sexualized arousal is almost always a factor in PE, it is by no means the only cause of the problem. Anxiety in its many forms rates a close second and, in some cases, is the determining factor in how readily the problem can be resolved.

Performance Anxiety: Normal Garden Variety

By far the most common anxiety experienced by men with PE, or with any sexual problem for that matter, is the fear of failure and consequently of being negatively judged—what therapists have termed performance anxiety. Unfortunately this simple phrase is devoid of the real potency of the feelings behind the words. By the time most men come to my office asking for help, they are experiencing so much nervousness around the issue of coming fast that the problem has become greatly exacerbated by the anxiety.

Many men, rightly or wrongly, believe that if they do not live up to the staying power they think women expect of them, they will be met with rejection or, even worse, contempt. The result is that by the time a man like this reaches the bedroom, he is such a bundle of nerves that he is far more focused on how he is going to do than on what's going on in his body. The by-product of this lack of focus is lack of control; after all, if he cannot monitor his physical sensations, how can be possibly know when he needs to slow down?

There are two signs that can help you determine if performance anxiety is a major factor in a man's PE problem:

- *The orgasms generated by high performance anxiety frequently lack the pleasure of other orgasms.* Many men have told me that their orgasms feel more like emissions that are not accompanied by a great deal of physical pleasure. Also, when performance anxiety is a big factor in the PE, men tend to come extremely quickly and sometimes for no obvious reasons. It is almost as if the actual amount of physical stimulation and pleasure a man is receiving were irrelevant. One described it this way: "It's like peeing in your pants, except that there is nothing to indicate beforehand that you have to pee." Said another: "The fact that I come when I do doesn't seem to be related to how turned on I am. It's more like a reflex that comes seemingly out of nowhere."

  Unfortunately, when a man loses touch with his body because he is experiencing terrible anxiety, his rapid ejaculation can become almost like a reflexive reaction. In this way he is similar to a child who is being potty-trained. If a youngster is very worried about having an accident, in all likelihood he will have an accident even before his bladder fills. If a man is obsessed with coming too quickly, he will have a rapid ejaculation even before there is much sexual stimulation.

- *The premature ejaculation becomes less severe as the man feels more comfortable in the relationship.* Quite a few men come much more quickly when they are in new relationships and think that they will be rejected because of their PE than when they are assured their partners will be there for them, PE or no PE. This pattern is particularly prevalent, I have found, among men who are somewhat shy socially and for whom rejection by women is already a big issue. You can be certain that performance anxiety is a significant contributing factor if you find that your partner's premature ejaculation seems less severe after you have been with him on a number of occasions or after assuring him that the relationship is not at stake because of the problem. In some cases, in fact, the premature ejaculation may cease to be a problem altogether, although more often it simply lessens in degree.

Of course, the opposite is also true: A man's PE problem is likely to get worse when a woman puts more pressure on him to perform. Unfortunately many of us do have a negative, critical attitude toward men with PE. As discussed earlier, many women misinterpret lack of control and feel exploited. But if we are honest, there is often more to it than that: As much as women say they want men to be vulnerable, we don't want them to have problems. There is something distasteful to many women about a man's having a sexual problem, a feeling that is communicated sometimes silently and other times straight from the hip. The bottom line is this: Men's performance anxiety is not all in their heads. The extent to which a woman holds a man accountable for his sexual problem is the extent to which she is likely to prevent him from overcoming it.

Consider Don, a twenty-nine-year-old male who came to me with a severe PE problem that he claimed was getting rapidly and progressively worse. At this point the problem manifested itself in his coming within twenty seconds after penetration. The situation was not always that bad, however. When we traced the history of Don's PE problem, it was obvious that he never had the greatest control. Although on occasion he said he could last up to five minutes with intravaginal thrusting, he would most often come within a minute or two of penetration. But there was no doubt that the state of his control had deteriorated since he started seeing Linda nine months before. "She is at her wits' end with the problem," Don told me. "I love her and want our relationship to work out, but now every time we make love, I feel like there's a guillotine over my head. I know that she'd going to leave me if I don't fix this thing quickly."

Not only does an attitude like Linda's make a man's PE problem worse, but in a frantic attempt to control their ejaculations under pressure, some men begin tuning out sexual feelings. Because a man may no longer feel any sexual pleasure, the result is not infrequently a full-blown erection problem. (More about this in the next chapter.) Clearly, if we want men to feel less performance pressure so they can overcome their premature ejaculation problems, we have to stop being catalysts for the pressure.

WHEN THE CAUSE OF PE
IS MORE DEEPLY ROOTED

When I first meet a patient with premature ejaculation, I generally tell him that if he has to have a sexual problem, PE is the one to have because it generally is not caused by some deeply rooted psychological problem that needs to be resolved first. There are, however, some exceptions.

Performance Anxiety and the Fear of the Critical Mother

There is a certain type of man whose premature ejaculation is caused by a kind of panic that is outside the realm of normal performance anxiety. I am sure you have heard the term "castration anxiety," and it really applies here. The cause of the problem, not surprisingly, is most often a critical, "castrating" mother figure who withheld love as a way of getting her own needs met. The type of fear of punishment or ostracism that a man like this experiences if he comes too fast is a replay of this early fear and nothing short of terror of something absolutely horrible happening to him.

Because of this enormous anxiety, such a man finds it almost impossible to relax and focus on what he is feeling in his body at any particular time. When he comes, it is not because he is necessarily turned on but because he panics. He is not unlike a young child who, afraid of peeing in his pants, ends up losing bladder control.

A hallmark of a man with this problem is a constant, unrelenting need for love and reassurance. And almost no partner can be understanding enough because he does not believe that a woman can really care for him. In his mind every sexual situation is a potential failure and a risk of rejection. This, of course, intensifies his anxiety, making his PE problem that much worse. That is why it is almost pointless to try to work on techniques to help this guy overcome his PE without simultaneously working on his relationship to his mother and women in general.

Sexual Guilt

A second, more insidious cause of premature ejaculation is extreme guilt feelings about sex. These usually emerge either when a boy has been sexually abused or when he is from a religiously orthodox background. When the latter is the case, the PE presents itself in a fairly typical way:

- *The lack of control is so extreme that it frequently prevents intercourse.* A man with this type of problem thinks he has an erection problem because he rarely is able to make it to penetration. What is actually happening is that intercourse creates such anxiety that he comes before he gets there or as soon as he gets there so that he can get it over with quickly. A man like this also tends to experience a lot of anxiety about having children. I vividly remember the pain of one Orthodox Jewish male who cried as he told me that his infrequent success with penetration was making him something of a social oddity. Unlike most other couples in his age-group and background, each of whom had at least one child, he and his wife had not been able to conceive during the four years of their marriage.

• *His feelings about sex translate to little or no masturbation or terrible guilt when he does.* Most men, with and without premature ejaculation, masturbate to orgasm throughout their lives. For the man whose guilt about sex is intense, even masturbation is a taboo. Therefore, either he does not do it, or when he does, he does it superfast. Both scenarios, sadly, set the stage for developing premature ejaculation even when he marries, has a partner, and is allowed to enjoy sex.

Once again, working through the guilt becomes an essential component of successfully resolving a man's premature response in these situations. And this, of course, makes solving the problem more complicated and long-term.

WHEN PE SUDDENLY APPEARS: THE EXCEPTION TO THE RULE

As I mentioned earlier, most men with PE have always had the disorder to one extent or another. There are a few exceptions to this pattern, however, that need to be mentioned.

There is the development of PE in later life, particularly when associated with an erection problem. Men who try to compensate for what they view as ailing erections often develop PE as a result of over-sexualized arousal and anxiety. Typically these men begin to ejaculate without full erections even during masturbation. Almost always, once the erection problem is resolved, so is the PE.

However, if your partner is neither old nor impotent and he suddenly goes from being able to hold off for a reasonable period of time to consistently coming too quickly, one of two things is happening. He may have had a problem with premature ejaculation that he overcame earlier, and the reemergence of a problem with control, even if short-lived, can trigger his anxiety and make control difficult once again. It is easy to determine if this is the case because with a little understanding and patience the problem usually disappears.

And what if it doesn't? Chances are good that your partner is angry at you for something and that your relationship may be in trouble. One of my patients, for example, a young attorney named Peter, came to me with an atypical presentation of PE. He had been in a relationship for one year, and except for the first few sexual encounters in which he ejaculated too rapidly, his control was fine. Seemingly out of the blue, he told me, he found he was unable to have good control with intercourse. Upon close scrutiny of his relationship, it was uncovered that Peter was not ready to make the commitment to marriage that his girlfriend Linda wanted him to. "I guess I just want out as soon as possible," he blurted in one session. It was a perfect metaphor for his PE. Once he ended the relationship, his PE problem completely disappeared.

If you find that your partner sometimes seems to have excellent control, but at others has very little, there may also be some unconscious factors being acted out in his quick ejaculation. Remember, a man with good control is more or less able to decide *voluntarily* when he's going to come. If he is angry at you, consciously or unconsciously, he may decide to be selfish and not bother having control. When a spouse has a bone to pick, he will tend to be less giving and cooperative generally, and that tendency carries over into the bedroom. Knowing that if he comes quickly, you will experience less pleasure or will become angry at him, this may be his way of letting you know that something is on his mind. When he is confronted directly, his typical excuse is that he "simply got carried away." The real truth, though, is that he is choosing not to have control and to ignore your needs along with it. (Bear in mind that this is not the same as the lack of consistent control displayed by a man who has had a chronic PE problem and who, in the process of resolving it, has not yet established a high degree of consistency.)

The ploy is destructive. If you find that you are in a relationship in which this type of "one day he has PE, one day he doesn't" is common, you need a marriage counselor more than you need a sex therapist.

TREATMENT AND PROGNOSIS

When we take into account the wide spectrum of causes of premature ejaculation, it is extraordinary that the success rate for treating the disorder is so high. In other words, if your partner has PE, the chances are excellent that he can overcome it—that is, if he (and you) are willing to work at it.

There are two main steps involved in helping a man develop ejaculatory control, and they are addressed in Part Two. Since a man with premature ejaculation tends to rush ahead mentally, the first thing he needs to do is to learn to relax and focus on the physical sensations he is experiencing in his body at the moment he is experiencing them. If, for instance, his penis is gently being stroked and he is simply able to respond to the stroking rather than to all that mental anticipation, he will feel some arousal but certainly will not be out of his mind with desire. Also, by getting acutely in touch with his level of arousal, he will begin to know when he needs to make certain adaptations to slow down.

The second step in developing better ejaculatory control is to desensitize a man to what can be a habitual, knee-jerk, and often anxiety-driven reaction to certain kinds of stimulation. For instance, as I discussed earlier, when he is coming right at the point of penetration, he needs to understand that it is not the intense stimulation but his anxiety and loss of focus at that moment that is making him lose control. Therefore, he can become desensitized by breaking penetration down into small parts: having his penis near the mouth of the vagina, penetrating just a tiny bit for a short period, and then inserting fully but without subsequent movement. If he repeats each step again and again, his anxiety will be reduced, allowing him simply to focus on the feelings in his body.

How easily the problem can be resolved and the length of time it will take, however, are other matters entirely. In order to make a reasonable determination about the speed of recovery and about a particular man's prognosis in general, a number of factors need to be taken into account.

How severe is the problem? There is a wide range of intensity of premature ejaculation. Some men ejaculate from kissing, even before their clothes are off. (Usually when the PE is this severe, the man is also having fairly frequent wet dreams in adulthood.) Others have fairly good control until it comes to receiving oral sex or penetration, at which point they lose it. And others have some control with intercourse although it is not as good as they would like. Obviously the worse the problem, the longer it usually takes to resolve.

How physically sensitive is he? A factor related to how quickly a man ejaculates is his innate sensitivity to physical stimulation. In discussing treatment and cure of PE, sex therapists usually fail to mention that men, even those who have good ejaculatory control, vary in their responsiveness just as women do. Although most men with PE can resolve the problem, the degree of control a man will inevitably have and how long and how much he will have to struggle to obtain that control can be affected by how easily he is physically aroused.

How long has he had the problem? It is true that as men age, their ability to arouse quickly diminishes, so that a man with mild PE at age thirty may not be very premature at age sixty. As a general rule, however, the longer that a man has the problem, the more difficult it is to resolve. That is because over time sexual response, just like other responses, becomes habitual. The result is that a man who originally failed to develop control because of extreme sexualizing or performance anxiety may, at an older age, not suffer from either, but his body is still responding reflexively to certain sexual stimuli—i.e., having his penis near the vagina.

Are there underlying dynamics, such as sexual guilt or excessive performance anxiety? Obviously, if the cause is deeply rooted, the solution needs to address the cause. While the overwhelming majority of men with premature ejaculation can be helped by following a behavioral course of therapy, those who have underlying issues that are triggering or exacerbating the PE generally need to resolve those problems before a behavioral approach will be of much use.

Is premature ejaculation his only sexual problem? If not, his problem will usually take longer to resolve. In the case of the man who is suffering from both PE and an erection problem, for instance, the erection problem will need to be at least partially resolved before he even attempts to work on the PE. Interestingly, some men who have PE also have difficulty reaching orgasm at times, making the treatment and resolution of the problem a lot more complicated.

How much does he want to solve the problem for himself as opposed to only for his partner? This is as important a determinant as any. PE, unlike erection problems, is not always a problem for the man who has it. Some men who believe that women really don't enjoy sex or who have partners who, in fact, do *not* really like sex, may believe it's fine to come in one minute. Others, never having experienced the pleasure of a slow buildup of arousal, think that orgasm is the only goal of sex and want to get there as quickly as possible. Still others think that almost all men come fast and don't view the quickness of their orgasms as anything out of the ordinary. Then, of course, there is the type of man whose controlling personality will not allow him to deal straight on with the fact that he has a problem.

Whatever the reason, if a man does not want to overcome the problem aside from his desire to get you to stop badgering him about it, it will be difficult for him to take the necessary steps to develop the control you would like him to have.

3

Erection Problems

I clearly remember the first patient I ever lost. His name was Bob and he had come to me for therapy because his penis was not doing what he thought it should do. He was a thirty-four-year-old architect. He sat and fidgeted nervously on the couch in my office, and the combination of his crew cut, his slightly pudgy face, and his whiny inflection gave him the air of a twittering little bird.

"Lately, when I have been with my wife, I have been losing my erection some of the time, and it is ruining my life," he told me. "I would almost rather be dead. I would definitely rather lose a limb. To tell you the truth, I can't think of anything worse," he said. He must have seen the startled look on my face because he added, "Well, if something happened to any of my children, that would be worse. But nothing short of that."

"What about if something happened to your wife?" I thought. I bit my tongue but couldn't help thinking that this guy sounded like something straight out of a soap opera. There were a lot of things I could think of that were a lot worse than a penis that occasionally went limp: cancer, starvation, the Holocaust. Sensing my disapproval, he suddenly got up, headed for the door, and then, turning around, looked me in the eye and said, "I know you must think I am being melodramatic, but as a woman you cannot possibly understand."

He was right. It took a long time for me to develop an understanding of what it must be like for a man to have an erection problem. As a woman I had no comparable point of reference from which to empathize. If I were unable to have orgasms, I could imagine feeling sexually inadequate, but I would definitely rather have that problem than lose an arm or leg. Not so for a man. A man's penis is really his fifth and most important limb. Lose a leg, and he cannot run. Lose his potency, and he does not feel like a man.

Erection problems humble a man. I have seen the inability to produce an erection on demand turn a macho gigolo into a nervous wreck. I will never forget Harold, a confirmed bachelor in his mid-forties, his gold necklaces sparkling against an open-collared shirt, his English Leather leaving its mark in my office for days, who broke into a cold sweat and nearly passed out at our first meeting when he told me that he had lost his erection with the last two women he had been with. Sounding like Sam in the television show "Cheers," he promised that he would swear off women, end his philandering days, and settle down with a nice Jewish girl, as his mother had always wanted, if only I could help him solve his problem. (His erections did return, and so, of course, did his womanizing.)

I have also seen a man risk his life rather than lose his potency. Recently a sixty-five-year-old retired accountant came to me because he began having difficulty maintaining an erection after undergoing surgery for prostate cancer. He fold me that he had rejected the hormone treatment that was his best chance for extending his life because his doctors told him the treatment could further affect his potency. "My wife is sixteen years younger than I am," he said with a desperation that was palpable, "and I do not want my hand and mouth to be my primary sex organs."

Even the veneer of the most obnoxious, controlling man usually cracks in the confessional of my office. Peter, a man in his early fifties, is a perfect example. Peter was a tough guy, from a tough neighborhood. While staring at my legs lasciviously, he told me that he had been having some trouble "keepin' it up" with his girlfriend for the past six months, professing all the while that "it really ain't no big deal." In the evaluation it emerged that when he was nine, a sixteen-year-old baby-sitter had tried to get Peter to fondle his penis. When I asked how the situation was dealt with, he became somewhat hostile and then, alluding to the nature of his childhood neighborhood, told me, "We took care of da guy, if ya know what I mean." His request for help was no more endearing. "So, baby," he said glibly at the end of the first session, "you think you can fix my dick?" When I told him I thought I could, his body sank back against the couch with relief. He broke into uncontrollable sobs that lasted five minutes.

Of course, with a man like this, one's sympathy can be short-lived because his tendency is to revert to his old sleazy style as a way of covering his shame. Pulling himself together after setting up his next appointment, he could not seem to control himself from commenting that I had "good tits." Sensing my discomfort, he said, "Don't get so bent outta shape. After all, I'm still a man."

His last words echoed in my head. Having an erection is, to most men, precisely what it means to be a man, leaving them open to panic the minute their penises are even mildly uncooperative. Ironically it is exactly this urgency that often turns a minor erection problem into a full-blown case of impotence.

THE PERFORMANCE-IMPOTENCE SPIRAL

By far the primary cause of psychological impotence in men is worry about having an erection. A man can lose his erection for all sorts of reasons. Whatever actually triggers the problem, however, the anxiety that a man develops around the issue is what keeps it going and over time can actually become its number-one cause. By the time most men reach my office, their anxiety is through the roof, a feeling that sends them spiraling downward into an abyss of greater anxiety and, consequently, a greater sense of failure.

I call this syndrome the performance-impotence spiral. A man may, for whatever reason, lose or fail to gain an erection on a particular occasion. Unless he has been drinking (after all, it is a well-known fact that alcohol and erections do not go well together, a fact that even most men accept) or is fairly secure in his masculinity, he starts to worry or, in some cases, becomes panicked. "What's going on here?" he asks. "This never happened to me before." Now he has this bug in his brain that his penis is no longer fail-safe, and he approaches his next sexual encounter with trepidation. "Will it work this time?" says the little voice in his brain. When he is actually in bed, he is less into what he is doing because he is more into monitoring the state of his erection. "Am I getting hard enough? Am I getting hard enough fast enough? Am I going to lose it this time? Please, God, don't let me lose it again!" And maybe he doesn't, at which point he sighs in relief that he has been able to perform adequately, even though he's been too busy thinking about his penis to have enjoyed much of what he has been doing. Then again, maybe he does lose his erection. Actually, unless he is able to dismiss completely the first episode of erectile failure as an insignificant fluke, chances are his anxiety will cause him to have the problem again.

Now he has more than one failure to grapple with. His state of concern intensifies, as does his penis monitoring. He starts to become obsessed with the status of his erection, sensitive to its every upward and downward turn. He may even start looking at his penis periodically to ascertain its present rigidity. His anxiety makes his erection fluctuate. Or he may even lose it altogether. He panics. Maybe he begins wildly fantasizing in an effort to save a losing battle. Whatever he is doing, he is certainly not experiencing the sexual pleasure of the moment. On the contrary, he is out of touch with the moment and out of touch with his body.

Not surprisingly the problem tends to get worse. After all, if he is too nervous to pay attention to what he is feeling in his body, he is not feeling sexually gratified. And what is an erection, if not a pleasurable response to pleasurable sexual stimulation?

With each progressive failure, the more nervous he becomes. This makes it even more difficult for him to enjoy himself the next time, and the time after that, and the time after that. The timing of his erectile failure starts to become predictable. He begins to anticipate failure at the point that he last lost his erection. Most often that point is somewhere before or right after penetration because men equate sexual performance with the ability to have intercourse. His anticipatory anxiety heightens, and he starts "choking in the clutch." He eventually reaches the point where anything vaguely associated with inter-course—getting or putting on a condom, a partner who is signaling that she is ready for penetration—makes him so nervous that his penis does an instantaneous shrinking act. Ultimately he may reach the point where penetration seems like an impossible dream.

For many men, things go from bad to worse. A man who is struggling with his erections often begins developing other sexual problems, such as premature ejaculation and loss of desire. Invariably he becomes depressed, at which point he either withdraws or becomes so agitated that he is unbearable to be around.

IMPOTENCE-PRONE PERSONALITIES

Certain types of men are more likely to become desperate more quickly than others. A man who is a worrywart will panic a lot faster than one who tends to take things in his stride. The good news is that this Nervous Nelly tends to fly into my office the minute he begins having a problem. The bad news is that he is so obsessed with his penis that it may be only a short time before he can no longer have a full erection, even when he masturbates.

A man who is a perfectionist and extremely performance-oriented is also likely to become gripped with anxiety when his penis fails to present him in a favorable light. His solution is to put more pressure on himself to get it up; this, of course, only makes the situation worse. Because of his intolerance of failure, it often doesn't take long before he begins hiding out and avoids having sex with women altogether. If you meet a man who is professionally successful and socially skilled but who darts from attractive women as soon as sex becomes an issue, the chances are a lot better that his penis won't perform than that he is gay.

Combine any of the above personality types with sexual inexpe-rience, and you have a definite recipe for failure. In addition to having his erection to worry about, he expends a lot of energy generally worrying about his sexual performance. The result is a man who enters a sexual situation with nothing but anxiety in his head.

While a man who is hyperanxious, extremely goal-oriented, or inexperienced has a particular susceptibility to developing a full-blown case of impotency after a few erection failures, just about any man who has a repeated problem getting or keeping it up will eventually develop an anxiety about his functioning. When it comes to the link between a stiff dick and a man's sense of his masculinity, no man is immune.

"When you've got a cock that works, you think about sex five percent of the time" is the way an attorney named Mike explained it. "When it doesn't work, you think about it ninety-nine percent of the time. This problem is taking over my whole life. I don't feel good about things anymore. I don't feel good about myself anymore. It's on my mind constantly." His feelings are reflective of most men with erection problems. A man with an erection problem does not simply think, "I have a sexual problem." He thinks of himself as an impotent man.

PREDICTABLE PLOYS FOR
UNPREDICTABLE PENISES

How do most men deal with the angst of his condition? The answer is, in a word, desperately.

The magic pill: The most common response these days for a man is to run to his physician for a prescription for Viagra.™ Even one sexual failure is enough to send some men clamoring for the blue pill that has revolutionized the way we think about male sexual functioning.

There is a lot of good news about Viagra. It is the treatment of choice for organic impotence. Viagra is wonderful for men who have hardening of the arteries, nerve damage from prostate surgery, or other physiological conditions. Since it is often effective, it can relieve the immediate and often paralyzing anxiety that a man can experience about losing an erection. Viagra has also alerted us to a critical piece of knowledge about male sexual response: men over a certain age need direct genital stimulation to get and keep an erection. Finally, Viagra has given worldwide press to male sexual problems. Suffering from ED, while still unpleasant, no longer carries quite the same stigma it once did.

But there are down sides to the Viagra revolution. It can have a number of negative side effects, including a flushed feeling, headaches, heart palpitations, and seeing a blue haze. A few men have died from it. Viagra has also been widely misused. I have seen scores of young men in their twenties and thirties who turn to a pill rather than deal with even one night of performance anxiety. This is problematic because Viagra can be tremendously addictive psychologically. In the past few years I have seen a new type of sex therapy patient. He is a young man who takes Viagra once because he is a little nervous, and finds that he is then nervous about whether he can perform without it. Before he knows it, he is twenty-five or thirty and popping a pill every time he has sex. At some point he wakes up to the realization that he does not want to take the medication every time he wants to make love. By now, however, he is so nervous about not being able to get it up without Viagra, that he develops full-fledged performance-driven erectile dysfunction.

Besides its addictive quality, Viagra has set a new standard in male sexual functioning. No longer is it good enough to get an erection sufficient for penetration. Men of all ages now want the same kind of erection they got when they were eighteen. With that goal, every man over the age of twenty is likely to feel sexually inadequate. And the more sexual self-doubt a man has, the greater the likelihood he will go to extraordinary, and possibly dangerous, lengths to perform.

Nevertheless, millions of prescriptions are written for Viagra every year, many of them for men who really do not need it. When a man feels his masculinity is on the line, he may find it preferable to take a pill that could potentially be dangerous to his health rather than try to overcome the problem once and for all with sex counseling.

A twenty-nine-year-old entrepreneur who had absolutely

nothing physically wrong with him explained that he had dropped out of sex therapy (which was helping him, by the way) in favor of Viagra-produced erections. "You are not in the position to know how I feel. I go from feeling totally inadequate to being a great lover. I mean, with this pill I am sexually sensational! I am able to have intercourse in six to seven different positions without losing my erection. I don't care that my erections are artificially induced. I don't care that I might become a Viagra addict. I only care that my problem is gone and that I feel proud of myself."

In hot pursuit of a hotter woman: While a certain type of man runs to his doctor for a pill, others run into the arms of another woman. If you have a partner who is having an erection problem and the two of you are not working on it together, there is a reasonably good chance that he is trying to work it out on the sly. Even if he responds to Viagra and is monogamous by nature, he may be driven to go to a prostitute or begin an extramarital affair in an attempt to see if a newer, younger, more responsive partner can bring him back to life. Sometimes these brief trysts may be successful and help restore his confidence. This is particularly true if the cause of his problem is a less than satisfactory relationship with you. More often the problem does not get resolved, leading him to try another tactic to deal with his ailing penis.

Sexual antics of mind and body: Another common response for a man with erection problems is to devise all sorts of ways that he believes will make him feel sexier in his mind. He may suddenly begin watching pornography on a regular basis. Or he may try talking dirty to you in the hope that this will stimulate him. Or he may begin fantasizing wildly in an attempt to keep his arousal up.

His desperation may also be evident in the way he makes love. Trying to arouse himself mentally, he is likely to touch you in a way that feels less sexual than grope-and-cope. Sensitivity to when you're ready for intercourse? Forget it. As soon as his penis springs to attention, he will try to send it in. Chances are that he will also try to get you to climb on top of him. That's because he's afraid that his erection will wilt away if he takes the time to maneuver his body into male superior position. (He may become condom-phobic for the same reason.) And if he does manage to get it in, any attempt to make intercourse last becomes non-existent. The longer he lasts, the greater his fear that he will go limp, so he tries to come as quickly as possible. The fact that he develops acute premature ejaculation as a result is of little consequence. There is no contest in whether a man would rather have PE or an erection problem.

Swearing off sex: Another type of man may suffer in silence and throw all his libidinal energy into work. If he is single, he may become an almost complete avoider of women. If he is married, he usually adopts this tactic because he is afraid of rocking the boat with his partner. Sadly this usually results in the pair growing farther and farther apart. And unless he is old and feels over the hill, a man like this usually begins looking for another solution.

When all else fails . . . my office: If a man had a foot problem, he would go see a foot doctor. But even though sex therapy is usually the treatment of choice for nonorganic erection problems, the idea of going for any kind of psychological help is so degrading to most men that I am often the last resort. Having an erection problem is so embarrassing for most men that I see them only when they have already done everything they can think of and their prayers have not been answered.

THE MANY FACES OF IMPOTENCE

Unlike premature ejaculation, the causes of erection problems are varied and range from the simple to the complex.

The Heavy-Duty Sexualizer, PE, and Impotence

Becoming aroused more from the mind than from the body, a leading cause of premature ejaculation, is also one of the most common and easily resolvable causes of erection problems. This is particularly true if a man is over thirty.

Here is how it happens. Arousal has two components: physical and mental. But some men, over a long period of time, develop a pattern of arousal based almost exclusively on the mental component of sex, forgetting that an erection is primarily a response to pleasurable physical sensation. Rather than feel what is going on in his body, such a man turns on mainly from anticipating, fantasizing, watching.

A telltale sign that you have a heavy-duty sexualizer on your hands is that he can't just lie back and passively receive pleasure. Without the mental turn-on of touching or watching you, he is stripped of the major source of his arousal.

A man like this may function just fine, in his younger years, when his penis is able to jump to attention at the slightest provocation. But as he gets older, getting and sustaining an erection just by thinking sexy becomes a physical impossibility. Here is where he runs into trouble. In time all this head sex makes him lose touch with his body. He may even reach the point that he cannot stimulate himself to the point of orgasm without using a sexual fantasy. Having lost awareness of what is happening in his body, he does not know how to feel the pleasure that comes purely from being physically stimulated. In addition, since he never required much physical stimulation before, he may not know to ask for it now.

Considering the sexualizer's mentality, it is not surprising that a lot of young men with premature ejaculation problems become older men with erection problems. Men with PE can also develop erection troubles out of well-intentioned but misguided efforts to correct their problems with premature ejaculation. It is not rare for a man who comes too quickly and is attempting to last longer to try to tune out his sexual feelings. Rather than think about sex, he puts his mind on work or the laundry or simply stares at the ceiling. The result is that he loses touch with the sexual experience all right. So much so that he begins having trouble with his erections.

Physical Problems

While some men have erection problems because sex is all in their heads, others have difficulties because they have problems in their bodies.

Erection problems that are physical in nature are rare in men under forty-five or fifty years of age. There are some exceptions, though. Men with diabetes, circulatory or neurological problems, or other serious medical conditions may have trouble with their erections. Also, many medications, including those used to treat high blood pressure and depression, can cause erection difficulties.

There is also something I refer to as the floppy penis phenomenon that can be present in a man of any age. These men are suffering from an arterial leak that causes the blood to run out of the penis much faster than usual. A man like this is fairly easy to spot because even when he has a relatively full erection, the base of his penis is floppy. Also, when he loses his erection, it dies on him almost instantaneously, rather than gradually.

Except in the most obvious cases, separating an erection problem that is primarily in a man's body from one that is mainly in his head is a tricky task. That's because even when there is a physical component to the problem, there is almost always an added psychological component. And often it is the mental element that carries the day.

The case that comes most quickly to mind is that of a sixty-four-year-old musician who was suffering from severe hardening of the arteries. This, combined with the medicine cabinet of drugs he was taking, was certainly, according to his doctor, the cause of his inability to sustain an erection with a woman. Maybe so, I told this man, who was more or less resigned to living out the rest of his days "sexually dead." But there was also the possibility that the main cause of his total inability to function was depression. As it turned out, I was on target. After we worked through this man's struggle to come to terms with getting older, followed by a course of fairly standard sex therapy, he was able to function with a partner about 90 percent of the time. All this after five years of not being able to have intercourse and only partial erections with masturbation!

In light of the interaction between body and mind, how, then, can you tell if there is a physical basis to your man's erection problem? You can rule out a physical problem if he is able to get an erection consistently when he masturbates. A penis that isn't working properly because of physiology does not consistently decide to become rock-hard when it is touched by one's own hand and then suddenly lose staying power when someone else is present.

Determining that there is something wrong with his anatomy, however, is more difficult. Here are a few guidelines:

- *He does not get a reasonably full erection even when he masturbates.* A man experiences less performance anxiety with self-stimulation than with partner stimulation. If he can't get an erection alone, there is a possibility that there is an organic component to his problem.
- *He does not get erections in his sleep or wake up with them.* This strongly, though not definitively, suggests a physical problem.
- *He does not get an erection with oral sex.* Many men find fellatio the most arousing form of stimulation. A lack of response to oral contact may be a sign of an organic difficulty.
- *It is easier for him to get an erection standing or sitting up than lying down.* This tells you that there is a good likelihood of a circulatory problem's interfering with his erectile functioning.
- *There is no pattern to when he gets or loses an erection.* The timing of his erections is completely unpredictable. Sometimes he sustains an erection with not much trouble, and other times he doesn't get much at all. Sometimes he gets an erection with masturbation, and other times he does not.

Even if you find your partner fits all of the above, however, the problem still can be psychological. A man can become so distraught about his inability to have erections that he can lose complete functioning and have all the symptoms of a man whose problem is organic. Therefore, a visit to a competent urologist specializing in the treatment of impotence is in order to determine the source of the difficulty. (Let me emphasize the word "competent." I have treated scores of men whose urologists did little more than test their testosterone levels and cursorily check their penile pulse before recommending Viagra or an alternative. A thorough exam should include a sonogram and a Rigiscan,™ a device that measures erectile activity when sleeping. For greater clarification, a doctor may also perform a test to more exactly measure blood flow.)

What if the problem is physical? In addition to Viagra, there are a number of alternatives. There is an effective vacuum device that can help create an erection but doesn't exactly do much for spontaneity. There are substances like prostaglandin and papaverine that a man can learn to inject directly into his penis. (No, it doesn't hurt, though there can be some side effects.) Then there is the penile implant, which requires surgery and should be used only when the other options are unsatisfactory. A urethral suppository called Muse™ is also a good choice for some men. Still, even when part of the problem is physical, seeing a sex therapist is often a good idea to deal with the mental aspect of the problem.

Deeply Rooted Problems

One of the most bizarre stories about impotence I ever heard was from Pierre, a man who came from a small island in the Caribbean. Pierre's sexual history was uneventful in his early years. He began dating in high school and had intercourse for the first time when he was nineteen. He had a few short-term, sexually active relationships. When he was twenty-two, a local girl fell madly in love with him. He liked her, too, but began pulling away when she made it clear she wanted to marry him. For a while she simply badgered him, refusing to take no for an answer. When he finally told her he wanted to call it quits, she went berserk, dumped gasoline on his house, and burned it down. It is now twenty years later, and he has not been able to get it up with a woman since.

While this is not exactly your typical case history, some sources estimate that as many as 5 percent of American men suffer from a chronic inability to get or keep an erection with a woman. Some of these men have never had intercourse because their penises go limp at the point of penetration. Others have, on occasion, been able to have sex on a hit-or-miss basis, but without any consistency. Still others have been able to function successfully with one or two partners over the course of their lifetimes, but not with anyone else.

A man with this type of impotence has issues that run deep psychologically. Occasionally, as in the case of our Caribbean island man, the chronic inability to have or keep an erection comes from a traumatic end to a relationship. Usually, though, this man's problems go way back into his childhood.

A history of abuse: Physical, sexual, or emotional abuse or neglectful relationships with one or both parents are a common cause of impotence. A man who has been hurt by his parents may transfer these feelings to his sex partner. His belief is that his parents have hurt him, so his partners will hurt him, too. The bottom line is that he becomes unable to trust anyone emotionally enough to share his body with her.

Jeremiah immediately comes to mind. An exceptionally good-looking man in his late thirties, he suffered from a life-long problem with erections. He was not very forthcoming about his past, and the roots of his troubles defied me until the end of our third session. As he was leaving the office, I gestured good-bye by patting his arm. This six-feet-two, 220-pound hunk of muscle lurched with such intensity that you would have thought I had shot him. In the next session he revealed that when he was a child, his father had repeatedly picked him up by his forearms and shaken his head against the wall because of Jeremiah's failure to do well in school.

The physical bruises from his childhood are gone. The emotional scars are not. A grown man, Jeremiah cannot be touched without feeling like jumping out of his skin. It is no small wonder that he can't keep an erection when he can't trust someone enough to touch his arm, let alone his most private parts.

The castrating mother: Another common cause of chronic impotence is a deep threat in relation to women and intimacy. And though I hate to blame it all on Mom, unfortunately she is often the problem.

Lenny Franks is a case in point. When I first started seeing him, Lenny was a thirty-nine-year-old man with a Clark Gable charm. He was professionally and athletically successful—every bit the epitome of a man's man. But underneath the composed veneer was a sensitive little boy who had been constantly criticized by his status-conscious mother, who was more concerned with what the neighbors would think than with Lenny's feelings. Her endless ridicule took its toll on Lenny's emotional development. Over many years Lenny became increasingly out of touch with his feelings. He lived his life as if onstage, performing to the hilt. And sex was the ultimate performance.

The result of these dynamics was an intense fear of intimacy and a paralyzing anxiety about sexual failure. Unable to share his vulnerabilities with a woman and fearful that all women would humiliate him the way his mother did, Lenny developed a pattern of chronically losing his erection before intercourse. The few successes he had involved women who were either intoxicated or half asleep, allowing his performance anxiety to dissipate enough so that he could have intercourse. But with the same partner awake and alert the next morning, his erections disappeared as soon as intercourse became imminent.

Fortunately Lenny was a trouper and committed to resolving what he called his erection problem but what was, in fact, an intimacy problem. For two years Lenny and I worked together, and the more he allowed himself to feel vulnerable and open with me, the more sexually functional he became. Although Lenny still prefers being with a woman whom he perceives as nonjudgmental, his erections are no longer thrown off by the slightest bit of criticism.

Erections, desire, and inhibitions: Finally, a chronic erection problem is often a symptom of another sexual problem. It is not surprising that a man who is trying to run from unconscious homosexual impulses, or who has an inordinate fear of intimacy, or who experiences a lot of guilt or disgust will have a penis that fails to respond. These men are discussed at length in subsequent chapters.

Whatever the cause, if you suspect that you are involved with a man with chronic impotence, you need to consider whether you are committed enough to him to go through what can be a long period of treatment. Just as these problems take time to develop, they usually take years of psychotherapy to resolve.

HOW WHAT YOU DON'T KNOW
CAN HURT YOU (AND HIM)

Fortunately most erection problems do not have such deep-seated causes. On the contrary, the most tragic fact about men with erection problems is that a great percentage of them would never have developed a problem if either they or the women in their lives had been more knowledgeable about and had more reasonable expectations of male sexual functioning. There is much needless suffering that occurs around the issue of men's erections, an angst and a despair that could often be completely avoided if we were well informed about male sexuality.

The extent of ignorance is so pervasive that it tells us just how biased our society is against compassion for men. Over the years I have found that there are a number of facts about male sexual functioning that, if well publicized, could probably prevent the needless worry that turns most of what starts as one erection failure into full-blown impotence. These facts fall into two categories: unrealistic expectations about masculinity and misinformation or lack of information about what constitutes adequate male sexual functioning.

"Macho" Men Who Aren't So Macho
but Who Believe the Macho Myths

While some men develop erection problems because they are out of touch with their bodies, there is a whole slew of men whose penises stop working because they are out of touch with what is going on in their heads. These men have bought lock, stock, and barrel into society's view that a man is supposed to function with any woman regardless of his feelings about her or his relationship with her. Believing that men are sex machines, such a man assumes that his penis should be ready, willing, and able whenever there is an available female in the vicinity and that he should perform sexually regardless of circumstances. Like the postman who delivers the mail rain or shine, he is unaware that illness, death of a spouse, divorce, or loss of a job can affect sexual functioning. He is not allowed to have a headache or a bad day.

This erroneous notion has all sorts of spin-offs, from the relatively benign to the truly neurotic, that can get a man in trouble.

- *A real man doesn't get nervous.* Except he does, particularly when he is with a woman he wants to please. Ironically it is not the nervousness per se that gets him into trouble. It is his feeling that he should not be nervous and needs to hide his anxiety that renders him impotent.

  The process goes something like this. A man meets a woman he would really like to impress. He becomes anxious about whether she will enjoy him sexually, an anxiety that makes his penis waver. Being a "stud," however, he cannot tell his partner that he is nervous nor does he rely on Viagra. Now he has two things he feels he has to hide: his anxiety and his unsteady penis. This makes it virtually impossible for him to focus on anything pleasurable, and the result is his worst nightmare come true: a penis that fails to cooperate.

- *A real man has a sexual radar: He should know what to do, when to do it, and where to put it.* There is no doubt that despite this age of sexual equality, a man is expected to be the sex expert. He is supposed to take the initiative and know exactly how to orchestrate the situation, start to finish. Unfortunately no man is a mind reader, so if he is not met with the response he anticipates or if things do not proceed without a glitch, he may become anxious and lose his erection.

  Although this can happen at any stage of lovemaking, it is most likely to occur at the point of penetration. I have worked with dozens of men who developed erection problems because they had difficulty finding the vaginal opening, particularly in the male superior position. Common to all was the notion that a man, even in the dark, should be able to take aim and fire his erect penis into his partner in one deft move, as if guided by radar. Sensing the need to ask his partner to help guide him in, as if he had some great male deficiency, a man like this will opt to hunt and peck for the vaginal opening. Unfortunately, if he doesn't find it fast, he usually doesn't have much of an erection left to use, once he does discover it.

- *A real man should be able to get it on with any willing female whether or not he is attracted to her.* Rather than acknowledge that he needs to feel some desire for a partner to function sexually with her, a man will often question his masculinity when he loses his erection, even if he is in a situation that he knows he really does not want to be in. This just sets him up for a greater likelihood of failure in his next sexual encounter.

  I remember one patient named Albert, a thirty-five-year-old stockbroker who actually became impotent because of his need to prove to himself that he could "make it" with anyone. His problem began a year before when he picked up a woman at a coffee shop, took her home, and then, after beginning to make love to her, realized that he did not want to be in bed with her. Obviously he lost his erection. But Albert fancied himself a stud. Rather than avoid women he was not attracted to, Albert went on a campaign to prove that he could have sex with anyone regardless of his feelings. For months on end he went out of his way to have sex with women he did not find particularly attractive. That is, he tried to have sex with them. In fact, he successfully reached intercourse on only one occasion. After months of therapy, during which he confronted his irrational need to be the best in bed and his erroneous notions of what it means to be a man, Albert was able to accept his need to be selective with the women he went to bed with and resolved his problem.

- *A real man should be able to get it up and keep it up even if his partner is unresponsive or hates sex.* A number of young men I have worked with developed erection problems in response to some pretty serious problems on the part of their partners. One young accountant's long-term girlfriend, for example, suffered for months with vaginismus, a disorder in which the muscles of the vagina contract involuntarily. As a result, penetration was difficult and often painful for her. Another equally intelligent young man developed an erection problem when he was in a relationship with a woman who did not have orgasms and made it clear she really did not like sex much.

Now here's the amazing part. Despite the sophistication of both these men, each thought that there was something innately wrong with *him*. The fact that it is psychologically normal for even the most virile man's penis to go limp when your partner is in pain or really wants to get it all over with never crossed either man's mind.

The partners of these men often do their fair share to contribute to this insanity. Almost invariably, when I work with a man in this situation, he tells me that his girlfriend blames him for the problem. Jack, a twenty-four-year-old computer programmer whose girlfriend didn't enjoy sex, for example, told me that she blamed him not only for the erection problem but for her inability to climax as well. The fact that she never had an orgasm in her life, even on her own, did little to alter her blaming behavior. Given the backdrop of society's idea that a man should be able to perform, regardless of whether his partner is sexually turned on, Jack developed a mental blind spot and failed to make the obvious link between her sexual problem and his limp penis. In fact, it was only after he broke up with this woman and discovered he had absolutely no problem with a more responsive partner that he came to understand the source of his difficulty.

- *A real man is not supposed to need to be in a committed relationship in order to function.* Yet this is a far more common condition for many men than you think. The reason that this need for commitment goes unnoticed is that the man who has this condition either is out of touch with that need or struggles desperately against it. Consciously he very much wants to sleep around, views himself as a ladies' man, and is usually completely befuddled when he has an erection problem. His unconscious script, however, is another matter.

The best example of this emotionally monogamous male who wishes that he were macho is Brent. An imposing man in his late forties, Brent came into my office crestfallen after having read a novel in which the protagonist was able to ride on a horse through a wide-open field while screwing a hot babe at the same time. "Why can't I do that?" he asked with dead seriousness and tears coming to his eyes. The reason he couldn't do that was clear to anyone who spent ten minutes talking to him about his sexual history. Brent had been reared in a very religious household. On numerous occasions before getting married, he had attempted intercourse and had failed each time. Once he married, his erection problems completely disappeared, only to return after he divorced his wife. And now, just as before, he found he was unable to sustain an erection with a woman he knew only casually and had no intention of developing a serious relationship with.

Brent's problem was obvious. He needed to be in a long-term committed relationship in order to function sexually. Unfortunately he, like many other men of his type, was unable to accept his own sexual requirements. Another patient who also needed to be in a committed relationship before he could function well sexually put it this way: "It's inconvenient to have to wait to fall in love. There just aren't that many women that I meet that I feel that way about."

Inconvenient or not, the man who does not listen to his penis usually finds that his penis does the talking for him anyway.

Men Who Are Ignorant about the Sexual Facts of Life and Have Equally Ignorant Partners

The mythology surrounding masculinity is second only to the ignorance about male sexual functioning, particularly after the age of thirty. The list of sexual facts of which people are oblivious is endless. Here are the most common ones that, if not recognized, get a man's penis into trouble.

- *Men over thirty need genital stimulation, too.* How would you feel if all a man did to arouse you was to offer his wanting naked body to you as he lay back waiting for you to begin stimulating him? Absurd as this sounds, this is not a far cry from what a lot of men expect from themselves and what a lot of women expect from men. It is no secret that most men enjoy being physically stimulated. However, many men as well as women are unaware of the fact that men over thirty often *need* to be physically stimulated.

  I am not saying that lots of men do not get spontaneous erections. But as early as in the mid-twenties, as men age, it takes the average man longer to get aroused. He is also likely to need more direct physical stimulation in order to get an erection as well as to sustain it. Arousal and erection are not one and the same thing. A man may be very aroused by looking at you or touching you, but for that arousal to translate into a full, sustainable erection, physical stimulation is often necessary.

  A man who is unaware of these normal physical changes is likely to become very distressed when his penis does not respond the way it used to. Accustomed to getting and sustaining an erection simply from the excitement of the moment, he suffers a rude shock when things no longer work that way.

- *A man does not need a rock-hard, perfectly erect penis to have intercourse.* As a man ages, the quality of his erections also changes. Not only does it take him longer to get aroused, but his erection may not be as rigid as it was when he was younger. However, this lack of a hard-as-steel erection does not make him any less able to have or enjoy intercourse.

- *Erections wax and wane during lovemaking.* It is normal for a man's erections to be more or less hard at any particular point during a sexual interaction. In fact, in a man over the age of thirty, this natural ebb and flow is likely to occur up to three times in every lovemaking session.

The lack of awareness about any or all of the above sexual facts of life has the power to send a man who is perfectly functional for his age spinning out of control down the performance-impotence spiral. Rather than understand that his body is changing and rather than adapt to those changes, the sexually ignorant male begins worrying about his adequacy, a worry that usually translates into an erection problem. He does not recognize that even though his sexual responses are changing, those changes are no more significant than getting gray hair or a few wrinkles. The more frustrated he becomes, the less able he is to enjoy sex in a relaxed way. And the worse his erection problem becomes.

You might think that providing a man like this with accurate information about sexual functioning would alleviate the problem. In many cases it does so with remarkable speed. However, good information about sexuality is difficult to come by. I have been astounded by how many male physicians, even urologists, seem to be uncomfortable with talking about sexual problems generally and erection problems in specific. And I have been shocked by how many physicians are completely misinformed.

One thirty-year-old patient recently told me that the urologist he went to spent two minutes listening to him, asked no questions, including whether he was able to get erections with self-stimulation, and wrote him a prescription for Viagra. Another fifty-year-old patient of mine who was able to have intercourse but noticed that his penis had lost a little of its rigidity went to a urologist just to make sure there was nothing medically wrong with him. Not only did the urologist fail to discuss the facts about aging sexuality, but he suggested that the patient immediately begin a regimen of Viagra before he lost complete functioning. Another patient, twenty-eight, whose impotence was completely anxiety-based, was told by a urologist that his erection problem was caused by an enlarged prostate. He was put on medication for three months, which of course had no positive effect whatsoever.

Even when a man receives accurate information about sexual functioning, the problem does not always go away. I have been struck by how many men resist accepting the facts about aging sexuality, endlessly comparing their sexual performances with those of twenty-year-olds. Even after functioning is restored and a man can see for himself that he doesn't need a hard-as-steel erection to satisfy his partner, it still often takes him months to work through these issues psychologically. And if he gets hooked on Viagra, he may never do so.

This can be especially true for the aging man who gravitates toward younger women. "Maybe a forty- or fifty-year-old woman won't have a problem with my penis," complained one sixty-two-year-old divorcé whose erections fluctuated occasionally. "But these twenty-five-year-old girls are used to something else, and they may not know that what is happening to me is normal for someone my age. So how am I supposed to compete?" Suggesting that he simply educate his younger partner, rather than take a pharmaceutical, usually falls on deaf ears.

A man does not have to have a young partner, however, for him to have a sexually unknowledgeable one.

How Women Can Cause Erection Problems

If men are oblivious of what constitutes normal sexual functioning after thirty, women are that much more so. A sexually ignorant man who pairs with an equally unknowledgeable partner creates a disastrous formula.

Female Ignorance

A woman who reacts to a nonproblem as a problem often creates a problem. I have had married women run to my office in fear of losing their husbands because they have noticed some fluctuation in their partners' erections of late or because their husbands' fifty-year-old penises are not quite as rigid as when they married twenty-five years ago. One woman was convinced her husband was having an affair because "I just can't get him hard the way I used to, no matter what I do." When I spoke to her husband privately, I discovered that, in fact, he *had* gone to bed with another woman. But it was not because he wasn't attracted to his wife. Rather, he had begun to buy into his wife's concern about his less than perfectly hard erection and wanted to see if maybe being with someone new could help him resolve his problem.

Still others relate early jitters in a relationship to a true problem, thereby creating one. Like her male counterpart's response, the most common female reaction to a man who loses or doesn't get an erection is to ask, "What's wrong with me?" Particularly in a new relationship, a woman is likely to feel either that she is not sexually attractive to her partner or that there must be something she is doing wrong or not doing. An ignorant or unsympathetic female can put added pressure on a man, turning a case of early dating jitters into a chronic impotence problem.

That is exactly what happened to George. When he first met Donna, he was so taken with her that he did everything he could to impress her. His anxiousness to please was so intense that his nerves got the best of him the first time they went to bed, and he was unable to consummate their relationship. George was upset enough without Donna's disappointment. "She just cried and cried," George told me. "No matter how often I told her that it had nothing to do with her, she just didn't believe me." That set them up for some real problems. "Donna made it her mission to give me an erection. The next time I arrived at her house she was wearing a sexy negligee, and there were lit candles and low music in the background. Ordinarily this would have been very exciting, but I felt so pressured to get it up that I couldn't respond at all." Donna became more frustrated, and George's intense anxiety spiraled out of control. It took him two months to have intercourse successfully with Donna. In the middle of one night, when she was fast asleep and taking the edge off George's pressure to perform, he was finally able to penetrate. Even after that, however, sex with Donna remained fraught with anxiety. Ultimately he ended the relationship, but the experience left its scars. George still gets so unnerved when he is first with a woman sexually that he is never able to have intercourse.

Sexually Selfish Women and Impotence

Although a woman's lack of knowledge can precipitate a man's erection problems, devastating results occur when a man and a woman develop a lovemaking style that is oriented toward the female's pleasure over a long period. I cannot tell you how many of my patients have described lovemaking that is, to all intents and purposes, so one-sided it is little wonder they can't hold erections.

Mark, a thirty-three-year-old father of three children, had not successfully had intercourse with his wife in almost six months when he first came to see me. When I asked him to elucidate the intimate details of his lovemaking, it quickly became clear why he was having a problem. "We start by hugging and kissing," he told me. "Then I touch her all over, and since she has trouble coming with intercourse, I usually give her oral sex, which she likes a lot. After she has her orgasm, we have intercourse until I come—or I guess I should say we used to have intercourse until I starting having this problem."

"It sounds great for her," I told Mark. "But what about you? Does she play with your penis? When you are giving her oral sex, is she reciprocating?"

Sensing where I was headed, Mark suddenly became embarrassed. "Actually she doesn't stimulate me too much. She might play with me a little bit when we're kissing sometimes, but not much. She doesn't really like to give oral sex, so I don't pressure her."

"How, then," I queried, "are you supposed to get an erection?"—a question for which Mark had no answer.

Jon, a forty-five-year-old stockbroker, described an almost identical pattern with one slight twist. Unlike Mark's wife, Jon's spouse could have orgasms during intercourse if she was stimulated sufficiently beforehand. Their lovemaking would start with Jon touching his wife all over, leading to her lying back so he could stimulate her orally, until she would be close to climaxing, at which point she would exclaim, "Put it inside me, *now!*" Without Jon's having received sufficient sexual stimulation, his "it" wasn't ready to go anywhere.

Then there is Marty's wife who doesn't like foreplay. "She doesn't seem to like touching that much. For her, intercourse is the thing, and after a little touchy-feely, she likes to get right down to it." Talk about sex on demand!

Oftentimes a man is initially a willing participant in this intercourse-oriented style of lovemaking, particularly in the early stages of his relationship, when it works for him, too. Especially when he is young, he may be just as happy as his partner to roll around a bit and stick it in. In his twenties, just seeing his partner aroused may be enough to sustain his own arousal. He is complicit in this lovemaking style—that is, until he can no longer function under its rules.

Mike, the attorney quoted earlier who said his impotence was ruining his life, told me that up until recently neither he nor his wife was into much foreplay. "Our sex life in the past has been pretty passionate" was how he described it. "Often I would come home feeling horny, I'd kiss her and she'd get hot, we would quickly tear each other's clothes off, and I'd enter. We would then have intercourse until she came a few times, and then I'd come. That was fine with me until I starting having this problem."

The problem, which in reality was nothing more than Mike's greater need for genital stimulation, due to getting older, began spinning out of control because his wife, Jane, assumed that her husband was no longer attracted to her. After he finally convinced her that this was not the case, she then began accusing him of having something wrong with him. Since Mike had never needed direct stimulation in the earlier years of their marriage, she simply could not fathom why he should need it now.

The result of all this misunderstanding was not only a broken penis but a broken man. Mike developed such angst about his erection problems that he started losing desire for his wife. This created a great deal of friction in their relationship. He became increasingly anxious, and by the time I saw him, he was having trouble getting a firm erection even with masturbation. He began ejaculating with less than a full erection, resulting in the development of premature ejaculation. Mike sank into a deep depression. Despite the fact that he had been to three medical doctors, Mike was convinced that he was dying of an undiagnosed terminal disease.

There are far too many such broken men whose problems could be averted if the women in their lives learned to recognize and respect the effects the aging process has on male sexuality. In fact, in all the instances cited above, the erection problems were reversed within three months or less once both partners were made award of the reverse sexism implicit in their lovemaking and were educated about normal male sexual functioning after age twenty-five.

I am not suggesting that the change was immediate or easy, however. Like men, women can be very resistant to learning the facts. The fact that men are not always able just to get it up so flies in the face of what we have always been led to believe—that men are always willing and able to have sex—that the truth takes some getting used to. As much as we complain about the insatiable male sexual appetite, there is another side to us that views his incessant desire as a compliment. The necessity to stimulate the genitals directly to get or sustain an erection can also be experienced as a blow to our egos; after all, shouldn't our mere presence be enough to get men excited? It was particularly difficult convincing Mike's wife, Jane, that he now needed to have his penis stimulated in order to get an erection firm enough for intercourse when for years this was not the case. For a long time she took this as a reflection on her desirability. In fact, it was only when she began stimulating her husband and saw that, lo and behold, as he relaxed, he began once again to have spontaneous erections on occasion that she was fully convinced that normal aging male sexuality, rather than her own aging marred by stretch marks, was the real culprit.

ERECTION PROBLEMS CAUSED BY IGNORANCE: TREATMENT AND PROGNOSIS

Considering how devastated a man feels when he suffers from impotence, it is amazing how easily the overwhelming majority of cases can be solved under the right circumstances. Like the man with premature ejaculation, a man with nonorganic impotence needs to learn how to relax and focus on the physical sensations he is feeling in his body. This helps reduce the performance anxiety that is a staple among all men with impotence, as well as gives a man a consistent, physical basis for arousal that he can count on. The feeling of mental turn-on that can produce a firm, sustainable erection in a man of twenty-five is no longer sufficient to do the job as he gets older. But if he can focus on good feelings in his body and receives adequate stimulation, he will learn to trust his body once again to respond adequately.

It should come as no surprise, then, that the prognosis for a man with this problem has a lot to do with the woman in his life. Your partner's chances of recovery are excellent if:

- *You are willing to reconcile your ignorance with the facts.* Since a great many problems are created by overreacting to or simply not knowing about the predictable, normal changes that occur in a man's penis as he ages, accepting the reality of sexual development can make all the difference in the world. By throwing out your unrealistic macho notions about erections and replacing them with a realistic view, you change the fundamental assumptions that got the two of you into trouble to begin with.
- *You are willing to be sexually giving and provide adequate stimulation.* If the problem is a need for more physical contact, the cure is simple enough. If you are too inhibited or selfish to give your partner sufficient genital stimulation, the problem is yours, not his.
- *You are able to have orgasms in other ways besides intercourse and do not feel that coitus is the be-all and end-all of lovemaking.* If a man can feel reassured that he doesn't need a hard penis to keep you sexually content, a lot of his performance pressure will be reduced. This naturally makes the chances for successful intercourse much greater.

If you can succeed in all the above but things are still not improving much, chances are good that there is a significant organic component to the problem. In this case, medical intervention can be of great value.

But don't be naive enough to think that any of these treatments can, in and of themselves, restore a man's potency. Erections are, for a man, as much a matter of the mind as of the body. A caring, educated partner is the best medicine.

4

Low Desire or
No Desire for You?

"She told me to go to prostitute, something I had absolutely no interest in, so I decided to see a sex therapist instead," said Jack, a fiftyish, somewhat depressed-looking man whose complete lack of attention to dress belies his wealth and status. "The fact is, I have no sexual desire for my wife or for anyone else, and that's how it's been for fifteen years. My wife is afraid of divorce because so many people in the entertainment business get divorced, but this is driving a wedge between us." When I asked him why his wife was not with him, he claimed that she was afraid of being recognized. My own hunch is that Jack's lack of interest is so upsetting to her she is afraid to confront it.

Mindy, however, is not afraid. Crossing and uncrossing her legs, she is as agitated as a live wire. "*He* thinks the problem is premature ejaculation, which *he* thinks is no big deal," she says accusingly of her husband, Ross, who has a stiff smile plastered on his face. "That's not the problem. It's more global than that. We've been married six years, and for the past three his interest in me has been almost nil. Nothing I do makes any difference. The last straw was when I surprised him and bought a teddy. When he came home, he looked at me as if I had gone off the deep end and said, 'What's *that?*' We're just at different places sexually. I like to make love to Mozart and candlelight. He'd rather screw to Ted Koppel."

Premature ejaculation angers and frustrates women. Impotence can be taken as a personal rejection. But no sexual problem makes a woman feel as threatened and undesirable as a lack of sexual interest on the part of her partner. Most of us have been conditioned to believe that men have insatiable sexual appetites so that when a man seems to have little desire, a woman invariably feels that something must be fundamentally wrong.

More often than not, she is right. As the result of our ignorance, we often misinterpret or overreact to other sexual problems, but when a woman takes to heart the message that her partner lacks sexual desire for her, her instinct is frequently accurate.

THE TRUTH ABOUT MEN WITH DESIRE DISORDERS

What happens when you undress a man who seems to be low in sexual desire? In a rare number of cases you will find a man who has little or no interest in sex, including masturbation, period. Simply put, he never has had, never will have, and doesn't care if he has sex or not. Somewhat more frequently, when a man has little appetite for sex, the source is a more generalized depression. Feeling blue, whether chronically or temporarily, seems to zap the sexual energy out of most people, as do many antidepressant and antianxiety medications. And of course, physical illness of any kind makes those amorous feelings fly right out the window. Not surprisingly, in these cases, when you deal with the root of the problem, his sex drive returns.

Most often, however, when you dig beneath the surface of a man whose sex drive seems wanting, you usually find one of two things:

- *He has conflicts about women, sexuality, or intimacy, or all of the above, that he does not want exposed.* These problems inhibit his sexual desire.

    or

- *He has no problem with desire in general but simply lacks or has lost interest in his present partner.* In other words, it is not an absence of sex drive per se but a lack of motivation to have sex with the woman he's with.

That is why, unlike men with premature ejaculation, impotence, or a general lack of sexual confidence, who frequently come for treatment of their own volition, men with desire problems are often dragged in by their partners. Deep down, most men who appear low in sexual desire for their partners don't have a lack of desire when it comes to their right hands or, in some cases, with other sexual partners, and they know it. They are fearful that within the context of therapy, their secret will be discovered.

WHAT IS DESIRE AND HOW MUCH IS TOO LITTLE?

It is important to define what a problem with desire means. Men, as well as women, vary in desire, sometimes from day to day and week to week. All relationships go through ups and downs, during which a man may feel more or less amorous. The whole idea of what constitutes sufficient desire also relates to the social climate. In the 1970s, at the height of the sexual revolution, a person who didn't have sex on the brain a good deal of the time might have been considered to have a problem with low desire. In the 1980s, with the rise in sexually transmitted diseases and the emphasis on upward mobility, it was considered admirable to sublimate sexual energy into making money. In the last decade or so, the attitude toward desire has been mixed. In many circles sex seems to be socially "in" again, and there are a multitude of articles and newscasts addressing ways to fit sex into the busy lives of working couples with children. At the same time Germaine Greer, now in menopause and midlife, is espousing the joys of life without sex.

How do you know when there is a problem of desire? At what point do we say that a man's lack of desire is too low? When is a woman's concern about her partner's interest really justified? In some ways it is easiest to define a loss of interest or low desire by talking about what it is *not*.

- *Low desire is not the same as an inability to function sexually.*
A lot of women fail to recognize a man with low or lessened
desire because they tend to equate the ability to perform with
desirability. That is often, however, not the case. While it is true
that some men with inhibited desire are unable to get erections,
many men with decreased sexual interest can still function.

I will never forget the look of utter shock on one thirty-
nine-year-old wife whose husband, during the course of a
therapy session, confided that she really had not turned him on
sexually for years. "How can that be?" she said, crestfallen and
shaking with disbelief. "We have sex once or twice a week, and
you're always hard."

"All that takes is a little bit of stimulation and a fantasy,"
he responded, angry that she had been so out of touch with him
as not to notice the qualitative difference in their lovemaking.
"But that doesn't mean I've been enjoying it."

- *Lack of desire is not necessarily related to lack of sexual
frequency.* Although there is a tendency, especially over time,
for a man with a desire problem to engage in sex less often, this
does not always happen. On the contrary, many men who have
lost interest in their partners have shared with me the fact that
they continue to initiate sex on a regular basis just to keep the
peace. "I haven't felt desire for my wife in ten years and have
been having extramarital activities for longer than that," a
forty-two-year-old man who recently made the decision to leave
his wife told me. "But I knew that I could go only so long without initiating sex before Leslie would suspect something was
up, so when necessary, I would make love to her. I approached
it like another household chore: something that needed to get
done and that I would do to get it over with."

Often, too, when a woman gleans that her partner is losing
interest in sex, she begins, sometimes without noticing it, taking
over the role of sexual initiator. And since a great many men
with diminished desire can still respond when approached
sexually, sex may occur as frequently as before, thereby mask-
ing the problem of her partner's deteriorating sexual interest.

Conversely, a decline in sexual frequency or initiating on the part of a man may not reflect a lack of desire. I have spoken with countless men who have plenty of desire for their partners yet who go through periods when the actual frequency of sexual activity is diminished because of stress, physical problems, or other outside interferences.

• *Lack of desire is not the same as avoiding sex out of fear of failure.* A lot of men with sexual problems stop initiating sex with partners not because they have lost interest but because they are afraid of rejection. "I have been married twenty-eight years, and I still get that feeling of arousal just looking at my wife," confided a man who recently developed an erection problem as the result of the normal physical changes that accompany growing older. "But I feel so emasculated by this erection problem that even when I feel like having sex, I tend to stay away."

In the same way a lot of single men who feel sexually inadequate do not initiate sexual activity with women who really interest them because they are afraid of being humiliated. In fact, whenever a woman complains that there is a man in her life who seems interested but has not taken any sexual action, she may discover (if she sticks around long enough for him to do something or if she herself does something) that his inaction is not because he doesn't want her but because he thinks he will not be able to please her.

• *Lack of desire is not the same as a discrepancy in desire.* This is an important point. Let's say that in your perfect world you would like to have sex five times a week. But let's say that in your partner's perfect world there would be sex only once a week. Does that mean that he's undersexed?

A lot of women these days seem to think so. It has been so drummed into our heads that men are the ones with the greater sexual appetites that many women immediately assume that a man whose sex drive is lower than theirs has a sexual problem. Often this is not true. Although a man may desire sex less than his partner does, it does not mean he suffers from a problem of sexual desire.

How can you tell if a man simply has a low baseline of desire rather than a desire disorder?

- *There is consistency in sex drive over time.* This is the best clue, although by no means definitive. A man who has inhibited sexual desire may, at the beginning of a relationship, have sex frequently in an attempt to hide his problem, but over an extended period, he will tend to initiate sex less often. So if, since the beginning of your relationship, his sex drive has been constant—that is, he initiates sex at fairly regular intervals— chances are good that he simply has a lower drive than you do. In making this assessment, though, you need to be fairly certain that he is not masturbating a lot or having other sexual outlets on the side.
- *When you and he have sex, he is passionate and uninhibited and experiences no sexual problems.* Have you ever met a slim person who does not have a voracious appetite but nevertheless truly enjoys food when he eats? The man who simply has less of a sexual appetite than you do is similar when it comes to sex: He loves it when he has it but just doesn't need it that often.

That is not to say that couples who are sexually mismatched do not run into problems—frequently they do—but once the problem is accurately identified as different sexual appetites, rather than a lack of interest on the part of one partner, there are many adaptive measures that can bring the couple's sex life into better synchrony. For example, many women with higher drives frequently ask their partners to stimulate them orally or manually to orgasm or to hold them while they masturbate. And of course, even though a man's level of desire might be less and he might not have initiated a sexual encounter at a particular time, a creative woman can often get a partner in the mood.

HOW TO SPOT A MAN WITH A DESIRE PROBLEM

If a lack of sexual interest can be but is not necessarily related to frequency of sex, ability to perform, or a man's baseline sexual appetite, how can you determine if there is a problem? There are a number of signs.

- *He experiences little or no arousal from touching you or from seeing you aroused.* A man with normal desire enjoys touching his partner and seeing her aroused, not just because he likes giving her pleasure but because it is mentally arousing for him. The man who has a desire problem, however, experiences little or no sexualized arousal. His touch may seem mechanical, almost obligatory, and his main motivation is to meet the minimum requirements of getting his partner aroused. As his partner you may think that he is sexually selfish and unwilling to give unless he gets. Some men, however, particularly those who are performance-oriented, may fake an interest in touching and be rather good in the partner-pleasuring department. However, since touching women isn't a sexual turn-on for them, in time their preference to be passive and receive usually emerges.
- *He is not a passionate lover. When he has sex, he functions but does not become involved.* Men with inhibited desire may make great lawyers, accountants, or dentists, but they are not terrific lovers. To the man with a desire problem, sex is more about physical release than about passion. As a result, there is an air of detachment in his lovemaking.

  Being on the receiving end, you are likely to feel when you are with him that he is not all there with you. That is because he usually is not. In order to deal with whatever is blocking his desire, he does one of two things: Either he focuses intensely on the physical sensations he is feeling at the moment, or he becomes deeply involved with a sexual fantasy. Both serve the purpose of helping him circumvent his inability to be aroused by the actual sexual interaction.
- *He is easily distracted.* Since he needs to "be somewhere else" in order to sustain his interest, anything that distracts him from the physical sensations or the fantasy quickly creates a loss of arousal. He may, for instance, become irritated if you talk or even moan at the wrong moment or if you change the stimu-

lation, even briefly, because your hand or mouth is tired or you want to change positions. A man like that is also susceptible of being distracted because on some level he wants to get away from whatever it is about sex that is making him uncomfortable.

- *He masturbates a lot more than he approaches you sexually.* This is almost a certain indication that something is inhibiting his motivation to be with a partner. Obviously he feels a physical need for sex. And just as obviously there is something blocking his motivation from initiating sex with you.

- *He does not initiate sex much or as much as he used to.* Although some men keep up the guise of interest and continue to approach their partners, many more initiate sex less and less over time. While a two-week hiatus is no cause for alarm, you should be concerned when your partner does not initiate for months or years on end or if you notice a slow and steady decline in his advances. Also, if he seems to have a chronic headache when you try to lure him to bed, something is likely to be amiss.

- *When you complain about your sex life, particularly about the frequency, he remembers having sex more often than you do.* One quirky yet powerful indicator of a man who is experiencing a desire problem is that he almost invariably thinks he has had sex more often than is the case. It is very common for a woman who suspects something is wrong to begin keeping tabs on the frequency of her sex life. Yet if she records that she and her husband have had sex three times in the past three months, he is likely to recollect that it has been at least twice as much.

- *In conjunction with many of the above symptoms, he either has a chronic problem or begins to develop an acute sexual problem, such as impotence or difficulty reaching orgasm.* While it is a good idea to ignore an occasional erection problem, particularly if your lovemaking is generally lively and regular, you should not ignore a man's inability to get an erection or have an orgasm when the other symptoms of a problem with desire are present.

By now you probably have a good idea whether or not the man in your life has a desire problem. But how can you tell if his lack of desire pertains to all women or if his low libido is directly related to you?

IF THE PROBLEM HAS ALWAYS BEEN THERE, IT IS PROBABLY HIM

Although there is no cut-and-dry rule, a man with a general problem of inhibited desire does not suddenly develop the problem but has always had it. If, except for a period early in your relationship with him, during which he may have feigned more sexual desire than he actually felt, he has always had a number of the symptoms described above, chances are he had the problem long before you came into the picture. For a man with this type of inhibited desire, the source of difficulty is not the woman he is with but his feelings about sex, intimacy, and women in general.

Although these problems are deeply rooted and not easily solved, there is an enormous range in severity. At one end of the continuum there is the man who is so inhibited that he tends to avoid sexual contact with a woman almost altogether. And when he does become sexually experienced, he is likely to have a host of problems with functioning both sexually and emotionally. This type of seriously inhibited man is discussed in detail in the next chapter.

More commonly a man with a desire disorder is able to function, at least with some women some of the time, but his level of enjoyment of sex, and sometimes his functioning, are diminished by what is usually an unconscious blockage. The inhibition is usually a result of one or more of three factors: a problem with sex and intimacy, an underlying feeling that sex is dirty, and bisexual or homosexual impulses.

When Low Desire Is a Problem with Intimacy

Many men with desire problems have trouble combining intimacy with lust. The result is that there is an adverse relationship between the two:

The closer a man gets emotionally, the less desire he feels. These men fall into one of two categories.

Men Who Fear Commitment

The primary characteristic of this type of man is that even though he claims to want a long-term relationship, he loses desire for a woman when the relationship becomes emotionally intense. If you get a glimpse of this guy's past, what you most often find is that he is the product of two parents who have painfully endured an unsatisfying marriage. Unfortunately the link between his parents' misery and his own fear of commitment is often unconscious. That's why his diminishing desire is as baffling to him as to his partner.

Roy, a police officer in his mid-thirties, comes to mind. He was madly in love with Belinda, his girlfriend of two years. But he claimed he just did not feel any sexual desire for her over the previous six months. After questioning him about any stresses in the relationship or changes in Belinda's physical appearance and coming up with blanks, I chronologically traced all his relationships since he was eighteen, when he first lost his virginity. What emerged was an almost predictable pattern of one- to two-year relationships, each of which Roy had ended for a hodgepodge of reasons: She didn't like the country, she wanted more kids than he, she was too moody, she got a great job in San Francisco and he didn't want to move, and so on. With Belinda he had not found such an excuse and therefore unconsciously devised one. She just, for some inexplicable reason, didn't turn him on anymore, and how could he live the rest of his life with someone he didn't find arousing?

If you are in a relationship with a man like this, you are best off ending it unless he is committed to long-term therapy to resolve his problem. You should be on the lookout if:

- *He has a history of short-lived relationships because he is unable to make a long-term commitment to a woman.* Often, he will tell you that he wants a serious relationship, but he just hasn't found the right person.

- *He has a penchant for intercourse doggy style.* While this is not a hard-and-fast indication, there is a striking relationship between the man who consistently prefers this position and a fear of intimacy. There is something about the lack of face-to-face contact and somewhat depersonalized nature of this position that he finds attractive.
- *He doesn't like to kiss.* Again, this is not a definite signal. Still, there is a tendency for a man who has a fear of intimacy to find kissing too emotionally intense. And since he feels threatened when he gets too close to someone, he avoids any activity that makes him feel that way.
- *He is very passionate, sexually and emotionally, at the onset of your relationship, but as soon as things become at all serious, his sexual interest in you takes a nosedive.* This pattern is a hallmark of this type of man and should not be ignored.

Men Who Can't Combine Love and Lust

By far the most common conflict that makes it difficult for a man to feel hot for the woman he loves is his inability to believe that good girls enjoy sex. Classically this is known as the Madonna–whore syndrome. Typically a man like this puts a woman into one of two categories: She is pure, marriageable, and motherly, or she is sexy and provocative. In a nutshell, if a woman is very sexual, he does not feel respect and love for her.

A man with this pattern is easy to spot.

- *If he is in a committed relationship, he does not feel much sexual desire, but he is turned on immensely when he engages in extracurricular sex.* This kind of a man often, though not always, is very emotionally committed to the woman in his life. At the same time he doesn't feel very turned on by her sexually. As a result, he does not initiate sex too much at home, and when he does have sex, he performs perfunctorily. With other women, however, he is another animal entirely: hot, passionate, and always ready to go.

- *He may have a chronic problem functioning with the partner he is committed to, but with no one else.* Although many men with this problem suffer no concrete problems with their partners, some have constant difficulties. One patient of mine, for instance, has suffered from a chronic erection problem with his wife but has not once had an erectile failure with any of his other numerous sexual partners.
- *His extracurricular sexual activities are numerous, varied, and of short duration.* To put it simply, he sleeps around with a lot of women but does not become emotionally involved with any of them, so you do not have to worry about his running out on you. Just as he is not getting sexual satisfaction from his long-term partner, so he does not look to have his emotional needs met by his sexual partners.
- *His lack of desire toward his primary partner makes little sense of him.* "My wife has a body that most men stare at," one thirty-five-year-old police officer told me. "But for some reason that I don't at all understand, I don't find Marisa attractive at all."

If you are this man's steady partner, it can be a little more difficult for you to spot the problem because he is not likely to share his passionate sexual flings with you. Nevertheless, there are some pretty clear signs that can help you determine if the man you are with falls into this category.

- *He looks at other women lasciviously.*
- *If you have daughters, he gets irrationally upset by the thought of their being sexual.*
- *He is embarrassed by or refuses to watch dirty movies with you.*
- *You are a woman who is sexually inhibited or uninterested or who does not have orgasms easily, and your partner does not insist that you do anything to change this. On the contrary, he may sabotage your sexuality in subtle ways.*

This last indicator is usually a surefire sign. A man who cannot combine love and lust almost invariably chooses a "good girl"—

someone who is not very sexual or is inhibited sexually—as a way of circumventing his problem. Of course, when you directly confront him, he will swear up and down that he wishes you were more sexual. He may even blame his lack of desire on the fact that you are not highly sexed or nonorgasmic. But upon closer scrutiny, it becomes quite clear that he considers you sexually safe and feels initially threatened by any attempt on your part to become more sexual.

David is a good case in point. When he first came to see me, he complained that he felt little sexual desire for his wife of three years and was recently beginning to have trouble ejaculating when having sex with her. The problem, in his mind, was that his wife was not a very sexual person and was unable to have an orgasm. When I suggested that he bring her in for treatment, he told me she would never consider such a thing. When he finally did confront her, he did so in a halfhearted way and backed off immediately when she told him she was uncomfortable with the idea. This was very atypical of David, who was more assertive in most other ways.

Unable to connect with the unconscious part of him that wanted his wife to remain asexual, that, in fact, had married her because she was sexually inhibited, David dropped out of therapy. He returned a year later in a panic after having contracted a venereal disease. After a number of months we spent exploring David's feelings about sex, it became increasingly clear to him that he thought deep down that sex was somehow dirty. Therefore, if his wife were sexy, she would be somewhat dirty. He began to realize that he had a stake in keeping his wife asexual and even remembered how early in their relationship he had become furious at her when during intercourse she had stimulated herself in an effort to become more aroused. His resistance to putting his foot down as far as her coming for treatment, he began to see, was really his way of sabotaging her sexuality.

Once David had worked through the conflicts he had about sex, his reaction to his wife changed radically. He was able to let her know in no uncertain terms that her lack of sexuality was a serious threat to their relationship. They started communicating more openly about her lack of orgasms and began working together to resolve this issue. And his desire for her, which had been absent since the day they married, began to emerge.

Not all stories have such happy endings because many men who have this sort of conflict do not come for therapy. If you have a sexual problem, then you might also be a saboteur when it comes to bringing the problem to a head. Just as men who are sexually conflicted marry inhibited women, so inhibited women tend to find sexually conflicted men. Particularly if he is having trouble functioning with you, it can be really easy to blame your problems on him and insist that he resolve his problem first. The result can be a long-term song and dance in which you both partake in keeping the song going. And unless the music stops, the problem will continue forever.

Inhibited Desire Because Sex Is Dirty

While the man with the Madonna–whore script can at least enjoy sex with women he feels are provocative, the belief that sex is intrinsically dirty or bad goes so deep for some men that they have trouble really enjoying it. This is particularly true when it comes to genital activity. A man like this is often stuck at an early adolescent stage of development. He is likely to enjoy and feel comfortable with kissing, light petting, nonsexual stroking—all the romantic aspects of sex. But as soon as you get down to the nitty-gritty physical level of sexuality, his body shuts down, sometimes to the point that he experiences serious erection problems.

This sexually immature and inhibited personality is marked by a number of characteristics:

- *He experiences an inverse relationship between how aroused he is and how sexual the activity is.* You notice he is very turned on while making out but gets progressively less interested as the touching gets more sexually explicit. The most extreme example of this type is a twenty-six-year-old man who told me he almost always had an erection when he was fully clothed and almost completely lost his arousal when he got undressed.

  Intellectually a man like this thinks there is nothing wrong with sex. But his penis tells another story. So do his fantasies, which invariably are more about seduction than about sexual activity.

- *He started masturbating at a late age or does not masturbate much.* Although other types of men with inhibited desire have plenty of desire when it comes to their own hands, the man who believes there is something bad about sex often does not enjoy masturbation either. In some cases he may not masturbate at all, or he started at a late age. (If a man has not stimulated himself to orgasm by the time he is fifteen, there is almost always something off about his sexuality.) Other times he may masturbate but does it "real fast and only for physical release when I need it," as one man put it. The natural urge for sexual pleasure is blocked by the enormous guilt that masturbation brings with it.
- *If he is single, he has an almost phobic fear of sexually transmitted diseases (STDs).* In this day and age it is foolhardy not to be cautious about sexual contact. But a man who is inhibited uses the fact that STDs exist as an excuse to avoid sex. No precautions, including testing and male and female condoms, are enough to allay his concern.
- *He may suffer from a chronic erection problem or extreme premature ejaculation.* Some men who believe that sex is dirty do not desire sex very much but are able to function. But when the bad feelings about sexual contact are intense, the desire to avoid sexual contact unconsciously translates into a penis that refuses to stay hard for penetration, or into a premature ejaculation problem that prevents intercourse from lasting more than ten seconds, or into an inability to come at all. A man like this shares many of the characteristics of the sexually inhibited male I discuss in the next chapter.

How does a man develop such negative feelings about sex? Frequently religious orthodoxy has something to do with it. Almost every religion has some serious prohibitions on sexual expression, and there is little doubt that individuals who have accepted these beliefs tend to think, on some level, that sex is not fun or natural.

Lack of discussion in the home about sex, interestingly, can have almost as negative an effect as explicit prohibitions. I have had many men tell me that the absence of sex as a subject of conversation gave them the feeling that sex was not a good thing. After all, if it were okay, why would everyone seem to go to these great lengths not to mention it?

Whatever the cause, the solution is rarely simple. Considering the depth and often unconscious nature of the problem, professional help is almost always warranted to overcome it.

Low Desire and Hidden Conflicts about Sexual Preference

Finally, a man might have limited sexual interest in having sex with a woman because he feels a strong attraction to members of the same sex. That is not to say that he is necessarily gay, although in some cases he might be. Just as often his sexual attraction to men is a result of his being blocked when it comes to allowing himself to feel attraction to a woman. That is because he may have buried sexual feelings toward his mother or sister that are forbidden.

In some cases the conflict is so intense that he completely avoids sex with a partner. (For the details, see the next chapter.) But in many instances he functions fairly well with a woman with the exception of his less than enthusiastic desire. True, he will not get turned on by touching her, but he is not necessarily turned off. And as long as the physical stimulation is pleasurable, and he can use his sexual fantasies for added excitement, he can lead a fairly normal heterosexual lifestyle.

Of course, if he is truly homosexual, there is always a chance that at some point he will come out of the closet. But often the attraction to men is less a physical desire than an eroticized emotional desire for affection from a man. If such a man has a powerful desire to live a heterosexual life, he can be very motivated to maintain an active sex life with a woman. And then a funny thing often happens: He eventually learns to enjoy sex more with a woman, although he never develops the kind of passion that a man without these conflicts experiences.

IF THE PROBLEM IS NEW,
IT'S PROBABLY YOU

While many men with inhibited desire have internal conflicts about intimacy, sex, or sexual preference, for many others a loss of sexual interest is due to circumstances in their current sexual situations. The best indicator that the cause of your partner's problem is on the home front is a slow, steady decline in his sexual interest in you. If at one time you had a reasonably satisfying sexual relationship but have noticed a distinct deterioration in the quantity or quality of your mate's desire, the problem usually involves you.

Not every instance of low desire is something to be concerned about. A loss of interest that occurs when a man is under a lot of stress at work or as a result of illness is usually nothing to worry about. These episodes are short in duration, and when the source of the stress disappears, the desire returns. But any loss of interest that lasts for more than a few months should not be ignored. A lack of interest that lasts for longer than that is invariably a signal that your relationship—emotionally, sexually, or both—is in trouble.

Sex and the Marital Battlefield

As much as we think that men will hop into bed with anything on two legs that is reasonably attractive, for many men sexual desire and intimacy are closely linked. I have worked with countless numbers of men who have shared with me the information that their wives are, in fact, physically attractive but that they have lost desire for them because of unsatisfactory emotional relationships.

- *A loss of desire can reflect deep feelings of resentment about a relationship.* A lack of loving feelings for his partner can zap the energy out of a man's penis. For many men who are monogamous by nature, the frequency of sexual interest is directly related to how happy they feel in their relationships. A man may even lose complete sexual functioning with his partner if the hostility runs too deep.

Interestingly, until his penis does the talking, a man may be fairly out of touch with just how dissatisfied he feels in his present relationship. Jeff, a thirty-year-old carpenter, is a good example of how the body can be the spokesperson for the mind. When Jeff first married Jenine, he was in love with her and very taken by what he describes as her exceptional physical beauty. But shortly after they married, Jenine's true colors as a criticizing and selfish woman began to show, and Jeff's sexual interest in her began to wane. Rather than see the red flag, however, Jeff attributed his loss of interest to the fact that the newness of sex with Jenine had worn off.

Over four years his interest continued to diminish, and he occasionally began having trouble sustaining his erections. But Jeff continued to convince himself that other things besides the relationship, such as work stressors, were at the root of his increasingly less responsive penis. This continued for five years, at which time Jenine announced she wanted a child. At this point Jeff stopped having erections almost completely, and he began to realize that his penis was telling him he wanted out of the marriage. Unfortunately Jenine got pregnant anyway on one of the now-rare occasions that Jeff could get to penetration with her. After their baby was born, Jeff tried to repair the marriage. But his feelings were too far gone. He began seeing another woman (whom he described as far less attractive physically but much more loving than Jenine) and left his wife shortly thereafter. "I felt terribly guilty," Jeff told me. "I wish I had stopped to listen to what my lack of desire for Jenine was telling me."

• *Men sometimes lose desire or withhold sex as a power ploy to punish their wives.* Women are not the only ones who get headaches when they are angry. Indeed, many a man unconsciously keeps sex from his partner as a way of getting even.

Richard, a dentist in his early forties, for example, came to me after a series of one-night stands about which he felt extremely guilty. Shortly before the birth of their fourth child, Richard ceased sleeping with his wife and began having extramarital liaisons. By the time he came to me for help, the sexual hiatus with his wife had been almost seven months long. In the course of therapy it emerged that he had not wanted a fourth child, a fact that his wife ignored by conveniently forgetting to use her diaphragm. Richard's loss of desire for his wife was an unconscious way of punishing her for her role in conceiving their child.

• *A man's other sexual problems can create such anxiety that he may lose sexual interest in his partner.* To rework the saying "Nothing breeds success like success," nothing leads to failure like failure. That is why a man who has a sexual problem causing a problem in his relationship may lose first the desire to initiate sex and eventually all sexual desire—period. One man in his mid-twenties, who had been married for three years, came to me complaining that he was experiencing almost no desire for sexual activity of any kind. In the intake, however, I learned that he had suffered from a lifelong and rather severe case of premature ejaculation, a condition that, despite his wife's lack of complaint, made him feel "like a sexual flop." Once his PE was cured, so was his problem with desire.

The situation is exacerbated if a spouse, out of either anger or hurt, lashes out verbally. One man, who had suffered from an increasingly persistent erection problem, says he lost all traces of sexual desire after his wife rejected a sexual advance, saying, "Why do you even want to do it when you do it so poorly?"

• *A dead love life can reflect an emotionally dead relationship.* Your relationship doesn't have to be hostile in order for your partner to lose interest in you sexually. Two people can, without rancor, drift apart over the years, and so can a man's sexual interest. The bottom line is that if you feel more like your partner's roommate than his lover, your relationship may very well be in trouble.

A business owner named Otto, who was convinced that he was sexually over the hill when he first entered treatment, became aware that his lack of response to his wife was a result of a marriage that had grown increasingly distant over the past fifteen years. "I perform," he told me, "but my mind is someplace else. I'm just not there. I don't enjoy it at all." When he eventually became aware, after engaging in extramarital sexual activity, that he was not dead sexually but that only his feelings for his spouse were gone, he asked for a divorce.

WHEN HE LOVES YOU BUT DOES NOT SEXUALLY DESIRE YOU

Of course, it is convenient and somehow infinitely less threatening to think that the relationship is at fault when the fire goes out of a man's appetite than to acknowledge that some men who love their wives nevertheless lose sexual interest in them. As scary as this is to women, it is nevertheless true that some men lose sexual desire for their partners even though they feel emotionally close to them. It would not be the whole story if I did not mention that some men I have worked with have confessed that their loss of interest in their partner is directly related to too much cellulite or too many wrinkles. As one seventy-year-old man described his lack of sexual desire for his sixty-five-year-old wife, "It just isn't fun making love to an old lady."

Another man whose wife had put on a fair amount of weight over the years confessed that "looking at her is a kind of turnoff." His solution was to "keep my eyes closed when I make love to her and pretend I'm with someone else."

But for the majority, when a man loses interest in his partner, it is not because of a few extra pounds or a few extra years.

The Signals a Woman Should Never Ignore

How can you tell if you are a woman at risk of losing your partner's sexual interest?

- *You have physically let yourself go.* Beauty is in the eyes of the beholder, and most men who love their partners do not lose their physical desire for them because of a few extra pounds. At the same time, more than one man has, albeit shamefully, confessed that dramatic changes in a partner's appearance can definitely put a damper on physical responsiveness to her. Men are highly visual, and when a woman puts on a great deal of weight or no longer takes pride in the way she looks, desire can be affected negatively.

• *You no longer think of yourself as physically attractive.* What can really put a damper on a man's sexual desire is his partner's negative feelings about her own sexiness. More often than not, when a man complains about his partner's physical appearance, it is less how she looks that is at issue than how she feels about herself. Maybe you feel less desirable because he has commented negatively on your appearance. Or maybe he has said nothing, but you feel upset about your weight or your flab or your wrinkles. Either way, the result is a vicious cycle: You don't feel sexy anymore, your partner picks up that message and views you as less sexy, and that lowers your sexual self-esteem even further.

One patient whose desire for his wife had been plummeting over a fifteen-year period described the cycle this way: "Nancy was never svelte, and she put on about twenty-five pounds after having our kids. Did it bother me? I suppose it did a bit because I remember urging her to go on a diet. Looking back, I probably should have kept my mouth shut because she started getting really sensitive about my touching her. She would actually slap my hand away from certain places, like her stomach, because she felt self-conscious about her love handles. To tell you the truth, I really didn't mind them all that much, but that didn't seem to matter. What did get to me, though, was that in time she began taking less care of her overall appearance. She just didn't make much of an effort to look good. She also started avoiding foreplay because she didn't like being touched, so sex became more and more mechanical. When we first met, we had sex regularly. Now it is rarer and rarer because I have reached the point that I'm not that interested anymore."

Another sixty-seven-year-old man who was married for forty-one years and had been losing his erections during intercourse for a number of months had a similar story. "My wife has put on about thirty pounds in the past year or two," he told me, "so when I look at her, I don't experience the same visual turn-on that I used to. But that isn't the real problem. What really bothers me is that since she's gotten heavy, she will only have sex with me on top. We used to use all different positions, but now she simply refuses. So I guess you could say that sex, or intercourse at least, has gotten boring." Fortunately, with a bit of prodding, this man was able to talk to his wife and enlist her cooperation in helping him with what he couched as his erection problem. As soon as intercourse became more varied, his problems with desire and erections disappeared.

- *Your own interest in sex has taken a nosedive.* Some women lose interest in sex for other reasons besides their negative feelings about their bodies or about getting older. Maybe you are angry at your partner. Or perhaps you are sublimating a lot of sexual energy into your children or your work. Whatever the cause, the less consistently amorous you feel, the less consistently amorous your partner is going to feel.

- *You do not have orgasms, or it takes you a long time to have one.* Most men say it is hard for them to get into sex if their partners do not enjoy themselves. And few men are naive enough these days to believe that a woman who does not consistently reach a climax is really having a good time. Eventually the inability to be responsive can have a tremendous impact on your partner's desire for you. Whether he initially ignores the problem or bends over backward trying to stimulate you to orgasm, he ultimately will lose desire unless you become responsive.

While the loss of desire is greatest with nonorgasmic women, many men have also told me that partners who are slow to respond can have a similar effect on their interest level. A fifty-two-year-old man who was very much in love with his thirty-eight-year-old wife admitted that even though he was attracted to her physically, the fact that it took twenty minutes or more of continuous manual stimulation for her to have an orgasm took a great edge off his desire. "There are times that I feel like my arm is going to fall off after we have sex," he told me. "And I guess that when sex becomes that much work, it takes a lot of the fun out of it."

- *You have ignored his grumbling, however faint, that he is dissatisfied with the quality or quantity of your sex life.* One of the saddest stories of a husband's loss of fidelity is that of Robert, a sixty-year-old married man of thirty years who had been unfaithful for fifteen. "I have had a lack of desire for my wife for twenty years," he told me the first time we met. "To me this is tragic because in all other ways she is my best friend." When I asked what he thought had happened, he told me, "The first five years of our sex life were pretty good in my mind, I guess, because I was so in love with her. But the familiarity made me desire her less, so I requested that we try other things. My wife is old-fashioned. She wouldn't have oral sex. She wouldn't try different positions. I told her on a number of occasions that I was dissatisfied with our sex life, but she just didn't respond. So I began looking on the outside, where I found women who were happy to do these things, and the sex was just more satisfying."

There is a great irony in this story: Robert's wife knew about her husband's dissatisifaction and could have remedied it fairly easily. "Do you think," I asked, "that if your wife had responded to your requests early in your relationship, you would be where you are today?"

His answer was an immediate and certain "Never. The truth is, I am basically a one-woman man."

- *You are not sexually innovative.* Even if your partner does not complain, if you do not work to keep your love life fresh, you are at risk of having him lose sexual interest in you. A lack of creativity and the unwillingness to experiment are the commonest reasons that men give for why they lose sexual interest in their partners. Although you do not have to engage in bondage games for most men to consider you versatile, men do like oral sex. And they do like having sex in different positions. And many of them do like to be surprised sexually. If you are inattentive to your sex life, you run the risk of losing your husband sexually to another woman who is more innovative.

Why Women Deny Their Sexual Relationship Is in Trouble

What is so astounding is that the majority of men who lose interest in their partners have told me that their partners seem oblivious to their loss of interest or stick their heads in the sand rather than acknowledge or deal with the problem.

Consider Jenine, the ex-wife of Jeff, the man I wrote about earlier who was so unhappy in his relationship that he eventually was unable to function sexually. Not only did Jenine ignore Jeff's loss of interest, but even when he lost his erection while she was trying to get pregnant, she apparently disregarded the significance of his ailing penis. "She spoke about maybe going for marriage counseling," Jeff told me when I asked what Jenine's response had been to his growing problem, "but that was the extent of it." In fact, when he told his wife he was leaving her, she was not only appalled but astounded. "She was incredulous. I know that I didn't want to face how bad things were, but until I split, she barely recognized there was a serious problem."

This story, with variations, is not rare. Richard, the dentist who had withheld sex for more than a year because of his anger toward his wife about their having had another child, told me that when he finally spoke to her about his loss of sexual interest, it was almost as if she had barely noticed at all. "I suppose it has been a long time, hasn't it?" was all she had to say. And Otto, the man whose relationship had died emotionally over many years, said that his request for a divorce was met with shock. "In her mind it seemed to come out of the blue. How could she not have noticed my lack of excitement when I was with her? How could she not pick up on the fact that I was a thousand miles away? How could it not register that over the past number of years she was the one doing most of the initiating? How could anyone as bright as she is be that dumb?"

The answer is that women, for all sorts of reasons, frequently ignore some fairly obvious signals that their sexual relationship is unhealthy.

- *Women indulge in wishful thinking.* We all tend not to see what we do not want to see and hope that the problem will magically disappear. Unfortunately this never happens unless a woman takes the appropriate action to resolve the problem.
- *Women often lack a real understanding of how important sex is to most men.* Sex is not as important to many women as it is to most men. Studies suggest that while women undoubtedly have strong sexual urges, the sex drives of men are more insistent and consistent, and most men do not take well to voluntary abstinence. A woman's sex drive, on the other hand, is more temperamental. Her desire is less intense, more sporadic, and more likely to be ignored if a host of conditions are not met, like being in the mood or being in love.

   As a result of this male–female discrepancy in sex drive, a woman may not really take to heart her partner's complaints about lack of sex or sexual variety. After all, if something is not that important to you and is not seriously affecting your feelings about the relationship, it can be difficult to understand how important it is to him.
- *A woman who never was interested or has become uninterested in sex may be glad no longer to be bothered by her partner's advances and may feel relieved not to have to turn him down continuously.* A few months ago I overheard a conversation at the health club where I swim. One of the locker room attendants, a spry lady in her early seventies, was complaining that her husband kept sexually putting the make on her despite her resistance to his advances. "At least he is still interested in you," responded the forty-fiveish woman she was talking to. "I wish he weren't interested," the older woman said nonchalantly, "because I have no use for that sort of thing anymore." Clearly, for a woman like this, a mate's loss of desire is not a source of concern but a blessing.
- *A woman who herself has lost desire specifically for her mate*

may view her partner's loss of desire as a way of getting her off the hook. Although we tend to think of men as the sexual infidels, I have worked with many a woman who, while sexually uninterested in her spouse, is getting it on hot and heavy with her lover. The fact that her husband is, in this case, initiating sex with her less and less frequently is a welcome relief. "The less I have to fake being turned on by my husband, the easier things are for me," one woman admitted to me.

- *Financial dependency makes a lot of women ignore and tolerate a lot of things from men.* Even with all these excuses, on some level almost every woman who is at all awake probably views a long-term partner's lack of sexual interest as an issue. If she is used to a particular lifestyle that she could not provide for herself, however, she might make a decision, albeit unconsciously, to live with the problem even if it means her partner has to go outside their relationship for sex from time to time. To the woman who is financially dependent, this may seem like a small price to pay for economic stability, particularly if she is afraid that her partner will leave her if she rocks the boat.

LOSS OF DESIRE AND INFIDELITY

Unless you don't mind if your partner sleeps around, ignoring the signs of loss of desire on your partner's part is a big mistake.

One of the truths about male sexuality is that when a man is unsatisfied at home, he is likely to look elsewhere. If he is not having good sex with you, he is probably having it with someone else. Of all the hundreds of men I have worked with, only a minuscule number are willing to live out the rest of their lives without positive sexual relationships.

Just how long a man will go without becoming sexual with another woman is difficult to predict. Some men I have worked with do not seem to wait very long before giving up on their present sexual relationships. Others go on for many years in unsatisfactory or nonexistent sexual relationships. One man, for example, stopped having sex with his wife in his forties and remained celibate for almost twenty years. Then, as he put it, "One day I woke up. I realized that I had no intention of living out the rest of my life without being sexual again." Still others continue to have sex sporadically with their long-term partners for many years until they finally work up the courage to become sexual with other women.

No matter how long they wait, however—months or years—at some point they almost all stop waiting.

5

Inexperienced Men,
Inhibited Men, and
Inhibited Ejaculation

A few years ago a friend of mine tearfully confessed that although she loved her boyfriend, she was having a lot of difficulty dealing with the fact that he came too quickly. In an attempt to assuage her anxiety, I assured her that PE was a fairly easy problem to resolve. "There are lots of problems that are a lot worse," I told her. "There are even some men who can't come at all."

"Now that," she said with a sheepish grin, "is a problem I wouldn't mind handling."

Her response, though understandable, was naive. Inhibited male orgasm (it used to be called retarded ejaculation) may initially sound preferable to a problem like premature ejaculation. Unfortunately a man who has difficulty coming usually has a host of other sexual and emotional problems.

There are some exceptions. Every once in a while I come across a man who is socially and sexually healthy except for the fact that he struggles to have an orgasm with a partner. Obviously there is some degree of inhibition there but nothing that cannot be worked out within a reasonably short time frame. Many medications, especially antidepressants, can have the effect of making it difficult for a man to have an orgasm. Also, a very small percentage of men who have difficulty or take a long time having an orgasm even with masturbation may have an organic disturbance of the neuroreceptors that lead to orgasm.

But in most cases a man who has trouble coming with a partner carries lots of other sexual and emotional baggage.

MALE VIRGINS

I will never forget the first adult male virgin I worked with. Twenty-nine, he had emigrated from France ten years before and had made a good deal of money in the import–export business. He was tall and graceful. He parachuted for recreation. His demeanor was assertive, almost aggressive. His combination of success, intelligence, and, of course, that irresistible French accent made him quite appealing. Yet there he was: a virgin. This man of the world had never even kissed a woman, let alone had intercourse with her.

This man was a walking paradox, a contradiction, much like the terms "masculine" and "sexual inexperience." The two just don't seem to go together. We have been so socialized to believe that men should be the sexual aggressors that we do not consider the plight of those who are not. But if you think that the sexually inexperienced male is an oddity, reflect on this: There may be almost two million virgins over the age of twenty-three in this country right now.

Approximately 5.5 percent of men in the United States fall into the category of "never married." Researchers believe that half these men are gay. Half of the remainder prefer the life of a bachelor. And stunningly, the other half are virgins! If you add the scores of what I call psychological virgins, men with extremely limited experience and even less confidence, the sum is no small number of men who fall short in the arena of sexual knowledge.

These men are heterosexually oriented, although some have homoerotic thoughts as well as heterosexual feelings. They often want desperately to marry and have children. Sadly they are sexually and sometimes socially crippled. And the older they get, the more crippled they become. What begins as simple inexperience can, if not resolved, become a tangled web of problems. Without the experience of being in a relationship, intimacy becomes an illusive and scary idea. In addition, the longer a man is alone with his fantasies and his own hand, the more difficult it becomes to have an orgasm with a real person of the opposite sex.

AT WHAT AGE IS VIRGINITY NOT A VIRTUE?

Nowhere does the double standard have a crueler twist. A woman who treasures her virginity in her twenties may at best be considered virtuous and at worst a little prudish. She may have some conflicts about intimacy or sexuality, but they do not stigmatize her the way they do a man. That is because once a woman is ready no longer to be a virgin, she only needs to give the cue, and there is likely to appear a willing teacher to help guide her down the path to sexual knowledge. It took one twenty-five-year-old sexually inexperienced patient of mine, who had a pretty face but was fairly overweight, a grand total of eight weeks to lose her virginity once she made up her mind that she wanted to.

A male in the same situation has a much more difficult road to travel. As I've noted before, our culture expects the male to take the lead and to be the more experienced sexually. So when he misses out on the normal courtship experience of the teens and early twenties, he usually runs into trouble. Ashamed of his lack of experience, he avoids women. The more he avoids, the more anxious he becomes, leading to more avoidance. Before you know it, you have a man who is headed into solitary sexual confinement. And unless he is seduced by a sexually aggressive female or gets professional help, he may stay that way forever.

MEN WHO SIMPLY MISS THE BOAT

What are these virgins made of psychologically? If they are young, it is often little more than an awkward adolescence marked by shyness and some conflicts related to body image.

You've Got to Be a Football Hero

Just as teenage girls are likely to harbor feelings of inadequacy if they fail to live up to the ideal of the cheerleader type, adolescent males also focus on their physical attributes as a way of measuring their attractiveness to the opposite sex. A socially shy teenage boy who also perceives himself as falling short in the looks department not only may miss the normal dating experience of adolescence but can remain stuck in the adolescent mind-set that says that physical attractiveness—not personality or financial stability—is the primary factor in being able to get a desirable female.

Richie, for example, was a twenty-four-year-old data processor who had been overweight as a child. In addition, his mother had always favored his two older brothers, leaving Richie with the underlying feeling that he was not quite good enough. Even though he now stood six feet one, was well built, and earned a decent living, he still felt inadequate, like the fat little boy he had once been. This feeling was coupled with a somewhat shy nature, which had prevented him from dating in high school, and a sensitivity to rejection that was reminiscent of his mother's early rejection. The result was that Richie missed both the social and sexual experiences he needed to develop feelings of sexual confidence. Now he was afraid that his lack of know-how would be the cause of rejection by a woman. He continued to hide out.

Men who are both shy and small in stature are ripe candidates for missing the courtship boat. Being short can be a devastating experience for a male, particularly during adolescence, when everyone, even the girls, are growing taller than he is. If a male is small and shy, the result can be a grown man who is convinced that his size is an unresolvable deficit.

Sean is a case in point of how the effect of being short can linger. When he first came to see me, he was twenty-four and a virgin. Sean was undoubtedly slight; he was five feet three although his body was perfectly proportioned. Although he was no Robert Redford, he was by no means unattractive. However, convinced that his height was preventing him from finding a woman he wanted to be in a relationship with, Sean was mentally stuck in adolescence. This became stunningly clear when I gave him the assignment of running a personal ad in the local newspaper. In his ad as well as in the telephone message he left for women responding to the ad, he mentioned his height first. Even more telling is what he failed to mention: the fact that he was a very successful art dealer and financially well off. When I questioned Sean about this omission, he seemed surprised. "I didn't know that money was so important to women," he said, a sure indication that he still viewed his own attractiveness by adolescent standards.

The most poignant case, and in many ways one of the most thrilling to see resolved, involved Dustin, a man who had missed the boat because of poor body image. Severely burned in a fire when he was four, Dustin went through his childhood convinced that he would never be normal. Yet, by his early twenties, after many years of painful surgery and facial reconstruction that occurred during adolescence, coupled with his ability to grow a mustache, Dustin looked normal.

Still, the scars of having lived through a childhood and adolescence of rejection by members of the opposite sex ran deep. It took many months of self-esteem building before Dustin felt comfortable just saying hello to a woman at the store or the bus stop on his way to work. It took him, given his devastating fear that a woman would say no, even longer to ask any woman to the movies. But Dustin has come a long way. He recently began dating a nineteen-year-old woman and had his first sexual experience with her. At twenty-eight he is accruing the experience that most males have when they are eighteen.

Fear of Commitment

Sometimes, of course, the reason for a man's lack of experience may go somewhat deeper. Some men avoid dating in their teens or early twenties as a result of having grown up with parents who were unhappily married. Associating dating with getting stuck in a relationship, a man from this background may not experience much interest in having a relationship. His virginity and lack of experience become excuses for staying away.

Remember the father and son I mentioned in the first chapter, the two who were patients of mine although both used false last names and neither knew that the other was coming to see me? This was the case with the son. While Dad struggled with an erection problem caused by his castrating wife, the son chose to stay away from women completely. When he first came to see me, he was twenty-nine and had never dated anyone more than four times. Even though he felt sexually attracted to women and was good-looking, he began to understand that he had chosen virginity because he was afraid of getting stuck like his father. He came from a staunch Catholic community, where divorce was frowned upon, and therefore believed that once he got married, he would be "suckered" for life.

Usually through therapy a man like this comes to see that his father's life is not his life. He also learns that his father had just as much a role in allowing the mental abuse to occur as had the woman dishing it out. These realizations liberate an otherwise sexually healthy male to become sexually active.

In this case I was able to do better than that. Well aware of the father's inherent inability to stand up to his wife and equally aware of his son's influence on his mother, I suggested that the son tell his mother that unless she stopped demeaning her husband and began acting civilly toward him, he was not coming home to visit anymore. The strategy worked. After a no-nonsense talk with his mother she agreed to a cease-fire. Seeing his father's situation ease gave the son the go-ahead to begin dating. And while the father, whom I still work with, continues to suffer from an erection problem because he knows that his wife prefers not to have sex with him, he has told me that his wife has been much less demeaning lately, although he does not have the foggiest idea of what caused the change.

Fear of Rejection

For other men, a hypersensitivity to rejection is what keeps them from gaining experience with the opposite sex. The sexy Frenchman I mentioned earlier falls into this category. His father had abandoned the family when he was a little boy, and since then he was terrified that he would lose anyone he loved. His fear was not of sex but of the dam of emotions that would burst forth if he became intimate with a woman.

Therefore, he opted for many years to throw himself into his work or pursuits such as jumping out of airplanes, just to prove how unafraid he was. By the time he was ready to make his foray into the world of relationships, he was twenty-nine and a virgin and had to deal with an image that suggested that he was anything but sexually inexperienced.

Although the causes vary, the difference between the male who has simply missed the boat and the man who suffers from much deeper sexual, social, or psychological conflicts is that the former usually finds a way to get the experience he has missed during his twenties. And once he breaks through the barrier of avoidance, his sexual functioning, although in need of some fine-tuning, is fairly normal. Perhaps he initially has a few fluctuating erections caused by nervousness or an inability to figure out how to penetrate. He is also likely to need practice in the area of partner pleasuring, although many of these men are avid readers and conceptually, at least, know more about female sexuality than do men with other dysfunctions. Occasionally, too, he may have a short-term problem with inhibited orgasm. But for the most part a man like this usually reports that if a woman notices his inexperience, she generally does not comment on it or reject him for it. (Whether this is a testimonial to the power of instinct, or the general lack of lovemaking skill among young men, or women's inhibition about expressing what they want and need sexually, I have not yet figured out.)

It is not unusual for the man who has missed his sexual adolescence to go on a sexual rampage once he has lost his virginity, trading in one partner for another in an effort to make up for lost time. I remember clearly, when I first began working with virgins, wondering if I had created a monster after helping Jerry, a striking-looking young man of twenty-five, overcome his social shyness. When I met him, Jerry was convinced that even though he no longer wanted to be a virgin, he wanted to have sex only with someone he was in love with. In time it became clear that this moral code was not really his but one that had been drummed into him by his mother, who had died when he was nineteen. Jerry, who described himself as always having an intense sexual interest in girls that he'd had to keep under wraps, thought that by allowing himself to have his own sexual mores, different from his mom's, he would be betraying her.

Eventually, as Jerry became an adult emotionally, he gave himself permission to develop values that he felt good about, including enjoying being sexual without having to be in love. I wasn't prepared for what happened next. By the time he was winding down treatment, this warm, kind, sensitive guy who had been concerned about not hurting the feelings of women had become a Don Jaun heartbreaker. His weekends were spent at singles bars, picking up women—sometimes he even managed more than one a night—and taking them home for sexual experiences. When I questioned this newfound promiscuity, he told me that he simply was into being "with as many women as I can just to see the difference."

Although I was less than thrilled by his behavior and about my part in creating it, I came to understand that for Jerry, as well as other late bloomers, this was a necessary step in reliving the adolescence he'd never had. He did get past it once the novelty of being sexual had worn off and eventually settled into a long-term relationship that, to my knowledge, he is still in.

Overall the prognosis is excellent, sexually and emotionally, for the inexperienced male who is still in his twenties and who more or less just missed the adolescent boat. Unless you meet him during his "making up for lost time" stage, you can be missing out on a good thing by rejecting a man because he initially seems shy and somewhat inexperienced.

VIRGINS (OR PSYCHOLOGICAL VIRGINS)
OVER THIRTY

The same, unfortunately, cannot always be said of the man who has not resolved his inexperience by his late twenties. Not only does his continued lack of experience create many more obstacles to overcome to become sexually functional, but he is also likely to have much deeper conflicts at the root of his inexperience.

How does a man get to be thirty plus and still be a virgin or close to it?

The Socially Inadequate Male

About one-third of the men I treat who are over thirtysomething and sexually inexperienced are paralyzed by shyness, lack of good social skills, and underlying feelings of inadequacy. Like the man who has simply missed the boat, he tends to be relatively free of sexual conflict and inhibition and can become sexually functional fairly easily—if he can get to the point of working up the gumption of asking a woman out and taking her to bed. Therein lies the rub. Unlike the man who has simply missed the boat, the socially inept male is plagued by a much more profound sense of social and emotional inadequacy.

- *He just seems, well, a little weird.* Not psychotic weird, but just off somehow. Being around him, you cannot help having the feeling that something is not quite right about him. Sometimes even the man himself is aware that there is something about him that people respond to negatively, yet he may be completely in the dark about what it is. That is because it is often elusive, hard to define exactly. The best way to describe it is a stiffness, a guarded unnaturalness with people. There is also often an incongruity in the person's body language—sitting in an "open" relaxed position with clenched fists, a smile that seems forced in light of the anger or otherwise pained expression in his eyes.
- *His general feelings of inadequacy are profound.* While there can be brief respites in his self-denigration, his underlying feeling is that he is a loser. Most often this self-loathing is the result of a dysfunctional family situation. One man, for instance, who was born thirteen years after the next-youngest sibling, described how his mother had always reminded him that he was an accident. Another told me how he had been hit on the head when he did not get good grades in school and subsequently developed a learning disability that further eroded his good feelings about himself. Whatever the cause, being around a man like this is uncomfortable because his negative feelings pervade his total personality.

- *There is often a history of substance abuse.* There is a very high incidence in this type of male of prior drug or substance abuse, including food. His shyness and low feeling of self-esteem are what lead him to abuse in the first place. However, once he recovers from the abuse, he not only is without the crutch of his drug but lacks years of healthy sexual and social interaction. Even if he has had some sexual experience, it is usually of little value to him because it was all "under the influence." As a result, he may have only a vague recollection of it and therefore has little confidence that it has taught him anything of value. The upshot is that he experiences himself as starting from scratch sexually.

What is interesting about a man like this is how unconflicted about sex he frequently is. Once he gets some sexual experience, his functioning is frequently normal and in many cases, according to the reports of these men's partners, better than average.

His relative lack of sexual hang-ups and inhibitions, however, does not eliminate the burden of his social and emotional inadequacies. Considering his exaggerated sense of shyness and underlying feeling of low self-worth, it can virtually take years before he develops the skills and confidence to go through the normal courtship process of acceptance and rejection required to find a long-term relationship. All too often he gives up before he gets there.

SEXUALLY INEXPERIENCED AND INHIBITED MEN

Although the socially inadequate but sexually unconflicted male is not uncommon, the largest group of virgins and psychological virgins in their thirties or older are men who appear socially "normal"—in fact, they are often educationally and professionally well above average—but who have deep conflicts about women and intimacy and are sexually inhibited and conflicted.

Men like this fall into one of two categories: the intact heterosexual or the heterosexual with homosexual imprinting.

THE INHIBITED HETEROSEXUAL MALE

This man has no conflict about his sexual orientation. He is attracted to women, and admires them from afar. His sexual fantasies are always heterosexual in nature. Unlike the conflicted heterosexual male with homosexual imprinting, the avoidance of sexual contact with a female has nothing to do with a lack of desire for women or sexual feelings toward other men. Rather, he has tremendous unresolved emotional feelings about and fears of women that inhibit him from pursuing an intimate sexual relationship with a member of the opposite sex.

Dennis is forty-five, outgoing, tall, slightly above average-looking, and well above average in intelligence and success. Up to two months ago he was also still a virgin. If you met him at a party, you would not have even the faintest idea that there is anything wrong with him, although in view of the societal taboo against never-married males, you might question his long-standing bachelorhood and wonder if he is homosexual. But Dennis is not gay. He has never had a homosexual experience, and his sexual fantasies have always been of women. However, Dennis has lived the whole of his adult life in his own painful emotional world—one devoid of close relationships with women, and men, for that matter—a world in which he fills the time with his career, his stamp collection, and his persistent and detailed sexual fantasies.

Dennis has spent a great many hours cultivating his fantasies by splicing together snippets of erotica he finds particularly pleasurable, creating, as he puts it, "the ultimate fantasy with the ultimate woman," providing him, when he masturbates, with "the ultimate sexual experience." He is not psychotic. He harbors great shame about these fantasies. At the same time they have provided him with a world without hurt and rejection as well as a way to escape his loneliness and depression.

Dennis, although somewhat older than most virgins of this type, is not atypical. He is successful professionally, has a perfectly normal social affect, and yet, because of many unresolved sexual and emotional issues, has never been in a sexual relationship with a woman. And although you would have difficulty detecting the problems that lie within when you first meet a Dennis or someone like him, a bit of probing into his history can give you some pretty good hints.

A Dread and Mistrust of Women

Almost invariably a man like this has a tremendous fear of, and often anger toward, women that comes from something having gone amiss in his early relationship with his mother.

Dennis is a perfect, although extreme, case in point. A few weeks after he was born, his birth mother left his father, his two brothers, and Dennis for another man. She was never heard from again. Dennis later learned that his mother had never wanted him. Impregnating his wife had been a ploy by his father to try to keep the ailing marriage together, a tactic that failed. How is that for role reversal?

Not only was Dennis out a mother, but his father didn't want him either. Inwardly he blamed Dennis for his wife's disappearance. He harbored a hostility that dug deep into his heart and later emerged in the form of unwarranted beatings. Also, Dennis's dad felt overwhelmed by having to care for his two other children. So two-month-old Dennis was sent to live with his aunt. He remained there for almost four years, and Dennis remembers feeling very loved and wanted. Then, for a reason that Dennis does not understand to this day, his father decided he wanted him back, and took Dennis to live with him. So now there was another mother gone, another attachment severed.

Dennis's father eventually remarried. Mom number three was a nervous, rancorous sort, although Dennis recalls a fondness for her. Maybe she was not the perfect mother, but she did, when she could, try to stand between Dennis's behind and his irrationally irate father. Dennis's father, through a combination of criticism and emotional abuse, beat Dennis's self-worth into the ground. His stepmother, while not the strongest person in the world, at least tried to pick up the pieces.

When Dennis was thirteen and entering puberty, his stepmother was killed in a car accident. When he most needed a stable female in his life to give him the courage to enter the heterosexual world, he was again abandoned. When she died, a part of Dennis did, too. Dennis retreated into his own private world, where he was in charge, where he called the shots—where no one could touch him. He had been hurt too many times, left too often, to risk that pain again.

Although Dennis's story is unique and more dramatic than others' stories, it is far from extraordinary. In fact, it is uncanny just how similar the backgrounds are to Dennis's of men who fall into this category.

- *He has an irascible, cantankerous mother.* Many of these men describe their mothers as having portrayed noxious images of being a woman: nervous, high-strung, and abrasive. Although intellectually, a man might acknowledge that all women are not this unappealing, emotionally there still remains a fear that he is going to get "stuck" with such a creature.
- *His mother is emotionally unpredictable.* "I just never knew what kind of mood she would be in" is the way one man described it. "One moment she would be loving and kind, and the next she would be critical and rejecting." These mixed messages, this emotional push–pull, create a situation in which a young boy, desperate for Mom's approval, is emotionally at the mercy of a woman's whims—a kind of perennial "she loves me, she loves me not" situation. The result is a man who needs the approval of women but retreats out of terror of not receiving it.
- *This unpredictable, untrustworthy mother dies, often at a critical juncture in his life, thereby abandoning him.* This is a fairly common experience among these men and exacerbates the already profound feeling that women can't be trusted.
- *He doesn't have any sisters.* The man who is sexually inexperienced and inhibited usually does not understand women very well. For many, that is a result of having grown up in a home without any women besides Mom, leaving him with the feeling that girls are somewhat alien. And what one is not familiar with, one tends to fear.
- *He is actually or psychologically an only child.* In other words, even if he has brothers or sisters, they are significantly older than he, rendering him alone to wrestle with his parents.

- *He has a hostile father.* Although this is not always the case, it is often true. As a result, a boy grows up feeling afraid of doing anything that might make his father angry, including being more of a man than his father is. This can translate psychologically into a fear of growing up and becoming a sexually active male.

Emotional Characteristics of the Heterosexual Conflicted Male

If the histories of men like these are amazingly similar, so are their personality traits.

- *He has an obsession with the physical attributes of women.* If there is any certain sign of your thirty-plus heterosexual psychological or actual virgin, it is a constant preoccupation with the physical appearance of the women he considers dating. Sometimes you may even catch him staring at a woman he finds especially attractive. Although physical attraction is important to most men, it is uppermost to this man. In fact, if you are not what society would consider well above average in looks, chances are you will never have the chance to become involved with a man with this background because he would never ask you out. And in the event that he did, he would end the relationship before it became emotionally serious.

    Since he is likely to be of only average looks himself, to say nothing of his sexual inexperience, you might wonder how he has the chutzpah to be so picky. In reality he is stuck at an adolescent stage of development when looks are everything. He does not have the experience of having learned that sexual chemistry goes way beyond pure physical appearance. In addition, his overall lack of self-confidence only increases his preoccupation with appearances.
- *He is cool and compliant on the outside, a volcano on the inside.* Another predominant characteristic that these older inexperienced and conflicted men share is a seething, unrelent-

ing anger that is hidden behind a superficial guise of niceness, sometimes to a fault. You are always walking on eggshells with this type of man, except that you usually do not know it until it is too late. In therapy a man like this begins by always being prompt for his appointments and never complaining about having to wait. He is deferential, agreeing with almost everything, and smiles even when it is apparent he is in pain. Then, one day, seemingly out of the blue, he either does not show up for therapy or leaves a nasty message that he has decided to end therapy, without any explanation why.

The problem is that this type of man is not only supersensitive but also completely inept when it comes to dealing with anger. As a result, he abruptly cuts off a relationship when things do not go his way because he does not know any other way of handling his rage.

- *He is a control freak and has difficulty dealing with not getting his way.* The combination of his infantile rage at not having received what he justly deserved and an adult life spent alone doing things only when and if he wants to makes it hard for him to compromise. He is used to being in charge, so any threat to this pseudo-independence is likely to be met with a great deal of resistance.

Sexual Habits of the Older Virgin

If the inhibited male has problems emotionally, he also has a number of sexual idiosyncrasies.

- *Late virginity:* This, of course, is the most obvious sexual aberration. Unlike young men who are a bit shy or who for other reasons have missed the opportunity for normal courtship of the late teens and early twenties, the older virgin has unconsciously avoided any opportunity to become sexual. That is why he ends up being as old as he is before seeking professional help. As ashamed as he is by his lack of experience, he is that much more terrified of having experience.

Unfortunately the lack of sexual experience with a partner creates certain patterns of sexual response that become problematic if and when he wants to relate to a woman sexually.

- *A dependence on masturbation:* While other men are engaging in sex with other people, the older virgin is engaging in sex with himself. And since this is the only outlet for his sexual feelings, he is likely to masturbate not only often but compulsively. Masturbation is enjoyable to most men. But to this man masturbation is not simply a pleasurable activity but a way of gaining emotional gratification and solace.

- *An addiction to a particular and often idiosyncratic way of masturbating:* The result is that a man becomes overly sensitized to the sensations he receives from his own hand, as well as to the perfect adjustments—faster, slower, harder, softer—that a person can get only through masturbation. He may also develop very particular types of motion, such as shaking his penis or tickling just the tip, to which he becomes responsive. He may also become used to masturbating by rubbing against a pillow or mattress. This is a sign of regressed sexuality as well as a problem in translating arousal to a partner.

- *An addiction to being alone with one's fantasies and lack of connection to another person:* Another factor that often makes the transition difficult from being alone to having sex with a real person is that for the whole of his adult life, a man like this has been arousing to a fantasy view of sex. Now, let's be clear about fantasies. The people in them are beautiful, or whatever the designer's image of beautiful is, do whatever their creator wants, and, most important of all, are nonthreatening because they never reject the fantasist. In a fantasy a man can do, be done to, or simply watch. Observing, in fact, is a common fantasy among men who feel sexually outside the mainstream. And the man who fantasizes can make this fantasy come and go at will. The result is a perfect, albeit noninteractive, sexual world that has little to do with reality and even less to do with the sexual and emotional interplay of actual lovemaking.

Sex after He Loses His Virginity

Considering his years of imprinting, it is little wonder that all sorts of sexual problems emerge once the older virgin takes the plunge and loses his virginity.

- *General lack of sexual finesse:* Although there can be a general sort of sexual klutziness, the lack of skill is most obvious when it comes to intercourse, particularly in the male superior position. These men frequently ask me, "How do I figure out where to put it in?" Older virgins have this idea, although I haven't the foggiest notion why, that a man, even in the dark, should be able to penetrate his partner in one deft move; that he should be able to take aim and fire his erect penis into the vaginal canal as if guided by radar. The words explaining to him that it is usual, even among sexually experienced men, for the woman to help guide the penis inside because the angle of the vagina varies from woman to woman are likely to fall upon deaf ears.

  Then, naturally, there is also an overall lack of ability that comes from lack of knowledge, coupled with some less than amorous feelings about certain female body parts.

- *An aversion to the vagina:* This is a staple among most men who have lived a life avoiding women sexually. It is true that we tend to fear things we are unfamiliar with. And to a forty-year-old virgin, the vagina, with its strange smells, textures, and hidden nature, is often a less than desirable part of the body. As one patient put it after I urged him to study a "beaver" shot at length in order to begin desensitizing him to his revulsion, "Well, it's not exactly made for aesthetics."

  The result is that particularly in the early states of his foray into the world of heterosexual sex, the virgin is likely to avoid touching the vagina or having oral sex. In some cases the aversion carries over to penetration, although his revulsion is likely to be less intense since he at least does not have to deal with the smell and can avoid some of the "sliminess," as one man described it, by wearing a condom. Still there is no doubt that a man with this history has a special sensitivity to the vagina's every nook and cranny—how bumpy, wet, big, or warm it is. And a man's preference to avoid this part of the female anatomy makes partner pleasuring difficult, to say the least.

- *Castration anxiety:* Another striking quality of these men is a very real fear of their genitals being hurt. This comes out in all kinds of ways. One man told me that he was afraid that his partner, who was slightly zaftig, would hurt his penis by bending it if she were in the female superior position. Others, convinced that women will inadvertently hurt them, complain of anxiety whenever their testicles are touched. Obviously, if a man is concerned with protecting his genitalia when he should be focusing on feeling good sensations, his pleasure will be compromised.

- *An inability to arouse without fantasy:* A common complaint among women who have had experience with an inexperienced man is that when he is making love, "he is not all here." That's because he is often deep into the fantasy he needs to get and stay aroused. That is not to say that he will always have to rely on fantasy for arousal. But it is difficult to erase the imprinting of twenty or thirty years without a protracted period of new imprinting to replace it.

- *Lack of sensation with intercourse:* The most common response I get from a man like this after he has lost his virginity is "Is that all there is?" In part, this is in response to the disappointment of discovering that the ceiling does not shake after the years of building sex up as something unattainable and otherworldly. But there is also a feeling that intercourse does not feel all that good, that there is not much friction. I call this the floppy vagina syndrome because so many of the men who have had this experience are convinced that the women they had sex with must have unusually large vaginas. In truth, the real problem is that such a man is so accustomed to the strong, perfect sensation of his own hand, or in some cases the feeling of rubbing against a pillow or mattress, that the feeling of coitus pales by comparison. Also, the sexually inexperienced man is often clumsy at intercourse at first and cannot coordinate his body to his best advantage.

- *Inhibited male orgasm:* As a result of his addiction to masturbation and his fantasies, his subsequent lack of strong sensation from penetration, and the underlying fear of intimacy that is commonplace among virginal men, inhibited orgasm is very common. The difficulty in climaxing is most pronounced with intercourse, although often a man like this has difficulty coming regardless of the type of stimulation in the presence of a woman—period. Not only is he unfamiliar with stimulation from another person, but he is also likely to develop a good deal of performance anxiety about how long it is taking him to reach an orgasm. "Is her arm, mouth, or pelvis getting tired?" he wonders. Naturally the more concerned he is about when he is going to come, the less likely it is that it's going to happen.

Can This Man Be Saved? A Prognosis

At this point you may be thinking that a man who falls into this category is a hopeless case and that pursuing a relationship with him is a hopeless cause. But this often is not true at all. Over the years I have seen men like these get married, and according to their wives, they make good husbands. So what should you do if you meet a man who tells you he has never been married and who you suspect falls into the category of the man I have just described? Should you write him off?

Not necessarily. If he has been heavily involved for a period of time in analytic psychotherapy and/or sex therapy in conjunction with a surrogate to work through these issues, he may be a reasonable candidate for a relationship, although if you meet him too early in treatment, he might not be ready yet. You will know if he has just recently begun to address these issues, as opposed to having resolved some of them, very easily. If he is early in the process, he will come right out and tell you. A man like this has a need to be totally honest right away about his lack of experience in relationships. A man who has worked through some of the barriers that have in the past prevented him from successfully pursuing relationships with women will not tell you right up front that he has zero or close to no experience (although if you start getting serious, he will tell you).

Also, he obviously has a much better chance of being a promising suitor if he is socially and professionally adept, but don't let the big bucks fool you. I have worked briefly with men of this type who are professionally successful but have extremely rigid and controlling personalities and believe that psychotherapy is something only for "sick" people. Individuals with personalities like this are difficult, to begin with. Lacking the normal relationship experience that most people have by their thirties or forties makes them impossible.

THE INHIBITED HETEROSEXUAL MAN
WITH HOMOSEXUAL IMPRINTING

The second type of the over-thirty virgin is the man who is primarily heterosexual in orientation but has some homosexual impulses to contend with.

How can you distinguish him from his hetero-conflicted counterpart? About half the time he has an effeminate affect, although this varies highly in its degree. At one extreme there is the guy you are convinced is gay, even though he is not. I distinctly remember having to bite my tongue to contain my laughter at my first meeting with Evan. Slightly built and sandy-haired, his voice lilting, he gesticulated rather grandly as he confessed that he "just could not understand why I don't seem to have a way with the girls." While he is usually not this obvious, often something in the voice or the gestures makes this man appear slightly effeminate.

Just as often, though, there is a complete lack of sexual affect; "asexual" is the word that comes to mind. He does not seem gay or straight, but more or less neuter. Unlike the situation of the heterosexual inhibited man who may seem shy but who nevertheless manages to sneak a peek at women in that typical male–female way, the fact that I am female and he is male seems irrelevant when we talk. There is a complete lack of sexualizing, often because he simply does not consciously feel sexually attracted to women.

Other times the attraction may be there but so deeply hidden that you would never guess it exists. One man, for instance, a well-to-do virgin in his mid-thirties, went from nerdy in appearance when he was glum to adorable when he smiled. Still, there was nothing in the least bit sexy about him. I had worked intensely with him for more than a year when one day, as we were discussing the type of woman he would find appealing, he told me that he found *me* attractive. I was amazed and thought that perhaps this was a positive sign of his coming out of seclusiveness. But further questioning revealed that he had been attracted to me since we had started our work together, had even fantasized about me. My jaw must have dropped in amazement because he was stunned by my apparent oblivion. "Couldn't you tell?" he asked, both hurt and confused about why his interest had gone unnoticed. But the truth was he had not given me the slightest glimpse that this might be the case.

If you cannot tell him by his cover, his fantasies are a dead giveaway. Virtually every man of this type I have ever worked with has conscious, recurrent homosexual fantasies. He often has heterosexual fantasies, too, but the mere existence of gay imagery when he masturbates has this man convinced beyond a doubt that he must be gay. After all, how could he imagine all sorts of sexual acts with a man and *not* be gay?

But he is almost invariably not homosexual. Go back enough in time, and you find that in elementary school he had the typical girl crushes that other heterosexual males have. But something usually happened around early puberty that prevented him from allowing his normal sexual interests to flourish, while at the same time encouraging desire toward males.

What kind of emotional backdrop produces a man with this heavy-duty confusion and conflict about his sexuality?

- *He has a very close, emotionally incestuous relationship with his mother that often, but not always, results from a physically or an emotionally absentee father.* In some families when there is no father or a woman feels emotionally estranged from her husband, she may turn to her son for comfort and closeness. A young boy may enjoy this special attention. He may even covet it.

As good as this intense connection feels, it becomes increasingly problematic. As a boy gets older and wants his freedom, he starts resenting his mother's reliance on him. Also, as he becomes aware of his burgeoning sexuality, the physical affection of a simple mother-son hug becomes laden with sexual overtones.

Now, what does an adolescent boy do, old enough to know that he is not supposed to want to go to bed with Mom, but with strong, uncontrollable yearnings in that direction? Particularly if the emotional boundaries between him and his mother are weak and his dependency on her is strong, he begins to shut down his sexual feelings toward women. The result is that this enormous faucet of heterosexual impulses, at their most pivotal point, is turned off.

Many men bury these feelings so deep that they remain forever lost. Even when their feelings can be retrieved in therapy, they are extremely threatening. That is exactly what happened to a patient named Gus. Even though there was little doubt that he had once had strong heterosexual feelings, those urges were arrested as a result of a sexualized relationship with his mother somewhere between the ages of twelve and fourteen. The fact that his sexual development stopped precisely around this time became humorously obvious when Gus started having sexual feelings about me. He would sit in my office like a dumbstruck teenager, staring, admittedly, at my breasts, then my legs—giggling, no less. When those adolescent feelings began translating into actual fantasies, however, Gus felt so threatened by what he considered "inappropriate" sexual feelings that he discontinued treatment.

- *He has a passive or rejecting father.* This is where the homosexual element comes from. Every boy needs affection and attention from his father, and when he does not get it, the

desire for male approval can become eroticized. Combine this
with the need to negate his heterosexual feelings, and you have
a situation that is ripe for the development of homoerotic ones.

- *He had a shy or awkward adolescence.* Many of these men
  describe themselves as having gone through a miserable gawky
  stage, marred by painful recollections of rejections by girls. Not
  surprisingly, the result is an ever-stronger desire to stay away
  from females and to seek out closer male companionship. And
  in light of the fact that during adolescence male hormones are
  pumping a zillion miles a minute, it is not surprising that sexual
  yearnings, even if not acted upon, can develop toward other
  males when females do not seem to be an option. These feelings
  are exacerbated when these pubescent boys, often for religious
  reasons, go to all-boy junior and senior high schools.

Put these elements together, and what you get is a male who is
confused, sometimes irretrievably, about intimacy and sexual preference. One of my saddest treatment failures was with a patient who had
this history. His name was Alan, and when I met him, he was in his late
twenties, had a successful accounting practice, and was a virgin. Two
years later he was no longer a virgin, but he still could not muster the
motivation to try to develop a relationship with a woman.

Alan was one of four sons, and he also had two sisters. Although
he does not remember his parents' fighting much, he does remember
his mother's continuously undermining his father for not making
enough money. In addition, Alan's father was fifteen years Alan's
mother's senior, so while Mom wanted to boogie, Dad wanted to sleep.
His mother's unhappiness translated into an overzealous relationship
with all her children, but most intensely with Alan.

By the time Alan was eight, it was obvious to him that his mom
preferred spending time with him to her husband, that Alan was his
mother's substitute spouse. At first, Alan remembers, he felt it was a
compliment to be "Mommy's best boy." But by the time he was ten or
eleven, he began to feel burdened by his mother's complaints about his
father. After all, he was supposed to be the child, not the parent.

The real breach with women came, however, when he was twelve or thirteen. His mother, while not one for parading around the house nude, failed to notice her son's normal prepubescent sexual interest in her. She made no attempt to cover up if her son was around even if she did happen to be in various stages of undress. As a result, Alan found himself masturbating to sexual fantasies about his mother. (Although many men with similar experiences do not consciously remember their sexual feelings before starting therapy, Alan did.) At about the same time the sister he was closest to, who was two years younger than he was, began developing breasts. So now he had not only one object of desire he felt ashamed about but two.

For all the emotional intensity Alan had with his mother, his relationship with his dad was devoid of feelings. If his father was too tired to be an active husband, he was also too tired to be a participatory father. "He was not mean to me," Alan recalls, "but he just never was there for me either." The lack of an adult male presence was exacerbated by his father's favoritism toward the oldest son. "He was always bragging about him, making comparisons between us. Nothing I ever did seemed to really matter to him, even though I spent my whole life trying to impress him. I studied hard in school for him. I went to college and became a CPA so he would be proud of me. But nothing I did really made much of an impression."

The blend of rejecting father and sexualizing mother, combined with a nasty case of acne and a flat-out rejection by the first and only girl he asked out in his teens, made Alan's adolescence a nightmare. He was extremely ashamed of his sexual feelings toward his mother and sister, and he felt completely unattractive to other girls. He was, however, popular with his circle of boys and formed tight bonds with his male friends. This pattern continued through his teens. In college he became especially close to one of his roommates, and on a trip to Florida over Christmas break, it became obvious to both younger men, neither of whom had ever had conscious homosexual feelings, that there were such rumblings between them. Alan never acted on these feelings, but they persist, to this day, in his masturbatory fantasies.

Alan buried his confusion in his career as an accountant for many years. But as he got older, the questions about his sexual preference greatly distressed him. In an attempt to make his foray into the heterosexual world, Alan went into a sex surrogate therapy program. It was there that he lost his virginity. It was there that he also learned that he could perform sexually with a woman, although, as he put it, "I was physically functioning but never really felt turned on."

The pattern continued in his few sexual encounters with women following the therapy. Not only did Alan not feel much excitement, but he began recognizing that he had some very strong negative feelings about having a close relationship with a woman. The one "long-term" relationship he allowed himself lasted only six months. He loved his partner, but the intense emotional demands placed on him by his mother, coupled with all the sexual conflicts he experienced, made the idea of a commitment completely untenable.

Alan and I were working on the sexual and intimacy issues when he lost his largest client and his accounting practice went under. He is now thirty-three, and whether I can help him if he returns to therapy remains unknown.

CAN THESE MEN EVER BECOME FUNCTIONAL?

Fortunately not all men in this situation end up like Alan. I remember the thrill of getting a wedding announcement followed a year later by a birth announcement from a man who, like Alan, had homosexual fantasies and was a forty-one-year-old virgin when we first began working together. However, because of the taboo on heterosexual feelings coupled with the homoerotic feelings, learning to enjoy sex with a woman can be a longer haul for such a man than for the man who does not have homosexual feelings.

In some ways both types of inhibited man are sexually alike after they lose their virginity. Both experience vaginal aversion, although it is generally stronger among men with homoerotic imprinting. Both tend to struggle with having orgasms with partners because of a long-term addiction to masturbation. And both, at least initially, suffer from a lack of sexual repartee.

However, the man with homoerotic imprinting has additional sexual difficulties to contend with.

- *Since he cannot give himself conscious permission to feel attracted to women, he does not sexualize.* Therefore, he gets little or no arousal from touching a woman's body. This makes it harder for him to experience desire.
- *He is more apt to numb out chronically during intercourse.* The inability to function—that is, to maintain an erection while claiming to feel little or no sexual sensation—is common among these men. Clearly, his body is feeling good, but the feelings are so forbidden that he cannot allow himself consciously to experience them. Once again, the result is a man who can function but does not experience much sexual satisfaction.
- *He does not allow himself to fantasize because of his guilt about the homosexual nature of his fantasies.* When I work with a man with any sort of inhibition, fantasy can be a blessing because it can help circumvent the anxiety. But more often than not, men with homosexual feelings refuse to allow themselves to use their fantasies because they feel perverted doing so. This makes it much more difficult to resolve their sexual problems with women.

Ironically, the man who learns to ally himself with his homosexual fantasies rather than try to squelch them has a much better likelihood of resolving his sexual difficulties than the man who does not. Sexual imprints are parts of us. When you consciously try to shut those imprints out, you shut out your general sexual feelings. The man who comes to understand that his homoerotic impulses do not make him homosexual, and who begins feeling okay about fantasizing about what comes naturally to him when with a woman, starts having some pleasurable heterosexual experiences. The fact that he is fantasizing about a man does not detract from the fact that in reality he is with a woman. So over time what develops is an increasingly positive attitude toward sex with a woman, which, with patience, can turn into actual desire. Not surprisingly, while his sex drive toward the opposite sex is on the rise, his homosexual fantasies begin to disappear.

Because of these added difficulties, the prognosis is somewhat worse for this guy than the heterosexual man with no homosexual imprinting. And if a man has crossed the line and has actually had a number of homosexual experiences, the task becomes that much more difficult.

6

Unusual Sex

"What is the strangest case you have ever seen?" a friend of mine asked as we sipped margaritas at a favorite Mexican restaurant.

I had to think. The first person who came to mind was a man in his sixties, adorned with rings on all his fingers and strings of beads around his neck, who came to ask me if I could help him rebuild his sexual relationship with his wife. For the longest time, he told me, he had been rather fond of being spanked with riding crops, of which he had a vast collection, while stoned on cocaine. His wife had no interest in these activities whatsoever, so he frequented a number of dominatrices for his spanking pleasures. Still, he claimed to love his wife and wondered if, at his age, it would be possible for him to learn to enjoy sex without being spanked.

Then there was "Jenny," who was six feet two, wore a tiny pillbox hat with a veil, twittered down the hall in spiked heels and off-black hose with a run in the back, and had the hairiest face I had ever seen on a woman. "She" chatted nervously for about ten minutes in a lilting baritone about "her" inhibitions and confusion about sexual matters. Suddenly "she" stopped and lowered "her" head shamefully. "I don't know if you've figured this out yet," she said, wringing her hands, "but the truth is, I'm really not a woman."

Then again, maybe it was Averill, an attractive male from Spain in his early twenties who, after spending the good part of one session staring at my legs, went into a trancelike state mumbling, "I can't help myself," and proceeded to expose himself.

As I mused through the list, and the look on my friend's face changed from curious surprise to utter disbelief, it occurred to me that over the years I had become immune to the "strangeness" of these cases. In fact, there are many more men with these disorders than most people realize. A recent women's magazine actually cited a study that reported that 11 percent of men have had an experience with fetishes, and 22 percent said they generally approved of them.* And while not my everyday type of patient, men with sexual preferences out of the ordinary were certainly not unfamiliar—to *me*, that is.

I emphasize the word "me," because men with behaviors that are out of the ordinary often appear to lead your average heterosexual lifestyle. Their diversions are almost always completely hidden from everyone, including their wives. Even when they first come in for therapy, they usually complain about erection problems or a loss of desire. It is only upon closer scrutiny that the real truth is told.

PARAPHILIAS AND SEXUAL ADDICTIONS

There is little doubt that our society is a sexually repressive and judgmental one, and what is considered deviant or abnormal behavior depends on whom you're speaking to as well as on the social climate. Up until the past decade, homosexuality was considered a pathological sexual aberration and listed in the diagnostic manual of clinical disorders as such. More recently, however, mental health practitioners have agreed that homosexuality is not a sexual disorder or perversion, although clearly there are still many people who believe this to be true.

Nevertheless, there are certain behaviors that raise eyebrows even among people who consider themselves open-minded about sex. These "kinky" or "bizarre" behaviors are technically called paraphilias. The

---

*Samuel S. Janus and Cynthia Janus, *The Janus Report on Sexual Behavior* (New York: John Wiley & Sons, 1993), reprinted in *Redbook* (March 1993), p. 70.

name comes from the Greek *philia*, which means "love," and the prefix *para*, which, roughly translated, means "out of the ordinary."

Paraphilias develop out of very serious disturbances in normal heterosexual bonding. Somewhere early in the paraphiliac's life, usually between the ages of three and eight, something creates a serious rift between love and sexual feelings. An event or series of events intervenes in the development of the normal boy-meets-girl attraction.

For instance, a boy who is sexually abused may become aroused when he is being exploited. As a result, he may grow up to experience sex as connected to abuse and completely separate and apart from love. Or a young boy who is being spanked may react by getting a panic erection, which is an involuntary genital response to fear. This can lead him to link pain or fear with erection. The result is that as an adult he may need to be spanked in order to get turned on.

You might think that a man with paraphiliac tendencies would be glaringly easy to spot. But he is not. That is because he often develops a double life as a solution to his sexual problems. A man may be a cross-dresser or exhibitionist who secretly acts out his impulses and then goes home and has sex with his partner. Then, when having sex, he replays the imagery of the ritual in his fantasy.

There is a wide range of paraphilias, including sadomasochism, fetishes and cross-dressing, voyeurism, exhibitionism, compulsive sex or male nymphomania, and coercive sexual behavior, such as wife rape.

But there are many other "odd" behaviors with which I have had experience. They range from the harmless, like cross-dressing, to the somewhat intrusive, such as talking suggestively for the purpose of making a woman feel uncomfortable. And a lot of what determines just how "weird" the paraphilia is depends on the partner. A number of women have told me that they have woken up in the middle of the night to find themselves spread-eagled and in the middle of intercourse. Some have said that they enjoyed this surprise and got into it. Others have told me that they considered the experience as nothing short of wife rape.

Regardless of what a partner thinks, paraphilias are problematic because they are frequently addictive. A sexual addiction is really a paraphilia that is out of control. Four main characteristics separate the paraphiliac from the sex addict:

> *The paraphiliac behavior is a necessary component for arousal.* While some men might enjoy particular behaviors that seem out of the ordinary, addicts need these behaviors in order to experience arousal.
>
> *Unmanageability and powerlessness:* Addicts cannot control their behavior even when there are grave consequences.
>
> *Lack of mutuality:* Addicts tend to impose their behavior on others even without their consent.
>
> *Shame:* Most addicts, even those whose behaviors are not extreme, experience a great deal of guilt and humiliation about their behaviors.

Paraphiliacs and sex addicts are tortured souls. It can be unbearable at times to do therapy with them because their pain is so palpable. Almost every man with these behaviors has a history of emotional, sexual, or physical abuse and frequently has been abused in all these ways. It is extremely common for a man who has been sexually molested to develop a sexual deviation, although it is almost as common for a man who has suffered extreme emotional abuse or neglect to become a paraphiliac.

There is general agreement that these out-of-the-ordinary practices develop out of fairly serious pathology, but no one seems to know for sure why one man becomes a voyeur while another becomes a male nymphomaniac. Sometimes the link seems clear. For instance, one patient who as a young boy became excited after exposing himself to a group of girls became addicted to exposing himself in order to become aroused. At other times, however, the connection between past history and the development of a paraphilia is vague at best.

As odd as it may seem, a paraphilia does serve a positive purpose. It allows a man who would otherwise be completely shut down sexually to remain sexually alive. As one forty-one-year-old man who was addicted to being spanked for arousal put it, "There is a powerful feeling of freedom of expression that I feel after these encounters. It almost feels as if my sexuality would have no outlet at all if it were not for this."

At the same time he is not oblivious of the stigma attached to such behaviors and his own shame. These practices are so far removed from average sexual behavior that these men are subject to extremely negative value judgments both from others and from themselves. "The exhilaration I feel after a spanking episode is always mixed with a profound feeling of shame," one man told me. "I know it is not normal. I know at this point I am not capable of engaging in an intimate, healthy heterosexual relationship. I would so desperately like to be able to do that, but at this point it seems out of the realm of possibility."

Although some paraphiliacs and sex addicts can and do recover, most do not.

FETISHISTS AND CROSS-DRESSERS

A fetish refers to the feel or smell of an object or a part of the body that has an almost superhuman erotic charge to it for a particular person. It is believed that fetishes often develop as a result of an early association of sexual arousal with a specific object. For instance, a lot of people think that the prevalence of foot fetishes and leather relate to a boy's having had an erection when near or in contact with his mother's feet or shoes or his own rubber diapers. Similarly, the desire to wear women's undergarments is thought to come from an erection inadvertently produced when a young boy tries on his mother's slip or panties. Fetishistic behavior ranges from what many people would consider relatively normal to the bizarre.

- *He insists you wear lacy brassieres, garter belts, sexy hose, and high heels.* We've all heard of men who are "breast" or "ass" men and of men who really enjoy watching their sexual partners dress in seductive clothing, such as lacy brassieres and garters. A lot of men like the excitement of seeing their partners dressed seductively, and if your lover buys you beautiful undergarments and asks that you wear them once in a while, this should be no cause for alarm. Although the desire to see a woman dressed this way can be considered a mild fetish, for most men it is not extreme enough to be considered a paraphilia. It also may be a turn-on for you to dress up in these outfits.

The difference between the man who enjoys seeing his partner in sexy garb from time to time and the paraphiliac is that your average joe does not require that his woman dress in this way in order to become aroused. Having you wear this clothing is not a necessary condition for arousal but an additional attraction. The more extreme fetishist, on the other hand, gains an almost trancelike pleasure from the fetish and may not be able to function without it. If there is coercion—either verbal or emotional—from your partner for you to dress in a specific way, you have good reason to suspect that his fetishistic impulses run deep.

Sometimes, because of a woman's own bias, telling the difference between normal male behavior and a more serious sexual problem can be difficult. A lot of women misinterpret the desire of partners to look at them in sexy clothing before lovemaking as an objectification. Usually this is not the case. Still, you should never engage in any behavior that makes you sexually uncomfortable. So if you and your partner are at odds about this issue, it may be a good idea for the two of you to have an open discussion with a sex therapist. Just as it would be unfair of him to make you feel inadequate for your unwillingness to engage in this type of sex play, so it would also be grossly unfair for you to assume that his desires are perverted.

• *He becomes aroused wearing women's clothing and women's undergarments in particular.* Known as a cross-dresser, he is a particular type of fetishist.

The first couple I ever treated after completing my clinical sex therapy training involved a cross-dresser and his wife. Sitting in my waiting room, they looked as Middle American as apple pie. She was petite, with gray eyes and a pixie haircut. He was slender and olive-skinned and quite handsome in a button-down polo shirt. They both were in their mid-twenties. I was nervous about my foray into treating patients on my own, and I signed with relief at how conventional they appeared. "Great," I thought. "It probably is a problem with PE. Or maybe she is having difficulty having orgasms with intercourse. Either way, no sweat."

My confidence was short-lived. "I love my husband, and I am happy with my sex life," the woman started. "It's just that there is one problem." Pause. "Paul likes wearing women's underwear when we begin making love, and well, it's not something that I am used to." So much for appearances. Paul confirmed his wife's statement, adding that his cross-dressing was something that he had tried giving up for years but with no success. He then went on to tell me that since his wife had trouble dealing with his need, he went away on trips where he cross-dressed, so that he had enough fuel for fantasy when he was with his wife. But now, he said, the fantasy was not enough. He needed to cross-dress to become sexually aroused.

The cross-dresser should not be confused with a drag queen. Although some men, particularly homosexual men, do dress up in women's clothing, they do not become sexually aroused by wearing the clothing. There are also some men who are confused about their gender and dress in women's clothing in an attempt to pass as women. For some, the conflict about being male is so intense that they go through the long and difficult process of having a sex-change operation. These men are transsexuals, or women in men's bodies.

The cross-dresser is different. The wearing of women's undergarments is an erotically charged event. Unfortunately, as with Paul, it is most often a necessary condition for arousal. One cross-dresser told me about an eight-year relationship of ecstatic sex with a woman who made no objection to his cross-dressing. Often they began an evening together by having dinner and with both partners aware of his wearing women's panties. Then they went home, and she assumed a dominant stance, demanding that he show her his panties. The situation progressed with continued mild verbal humiliation, leading to what was a passionate experience for both partners. When the relationship ended, however, he experienced chronic erection problems with other partners who did not know about or did not allow his cross-dressing.

It is this "addiction" that makes cross-dressing so problematic. In and of itself cross-dressing is benign. It hurts no one. It is not exploitative. The problem is that most women get turned off by the idea of a man in a teddy. And because of society's negative view of such behavior, the man who needs to cross-dress usually feels a great deal of shame.

- *He gets turned on by things that most people consider totally disgusting, such as enemas, feces, etc.* Okay. This is a subject that most people don't even want to think about, much less talk about. It is important for you to know, however, that there are some men who need to have contact with certain bodily secretions in order to have orgasms. Early experiences in their histories have made this strange link between what most people consider filthy and the erotic. Getting an enema or contact with these excretions is a substitute for normalized foreplay and intercourse.

THE VOYEUR

In one of the opening snippets to the old television series *The Odd Couple*, Oscar nearly gets hit by a car when he turns around to stare at a curvaceous figure while crossing the street. Millions of men read girlie magazines each month as well as rent X-rated videos for their viewing pleasure. There is no doubt that men like to look at women, and they do it whenever and as often as they can.

Does this mean that all men are voyeurs? Hardly. The thrill for the voyeur rests primarily in the intensity of sexualization, its illicitness, and fear of being discovered.

Voyeurism can develop in a relatively innocent way. A young boy may, for instance, see a woman undressing through his bedroom window and become aroused. He then may begin to seek out similar experiences to feel aroused. Fundamentally, though, voyeurism is sexual excitement at a distance. You can almost always tell a voyeur by his fantasies. Invariably they involve watching rather than doing.

Voyeuristic behavior ranges from the relatively benign to the addictive.

- *He enjoys watching you undress in a way that feels less appreciative of your body than lewd and oversexualized.* There is evidence to suggest that men are much more dependent on sight for their arousal than women are, and for many men, observing a woman in various stages of undressing can be a great turn-on. So, if he watches you undress in a loving, nonintrusive way but you feel uncomfortable, it may be your problem. Perhaps you are self-conscious about your body or are otherwise sexually inhibited.

  Being watched by a voyeur is a different experience. There is a coercive and insistent quality to his need to watch. You are also likely to feel depersonalized and violated. When you explain how you are feeling, he is likely to respond in one of two ways. He might be totally embarrassed and honestly tell you that he has been oblivious of his behavior. If this is the case, the likelihood of his being an addicted voyeur is slim. On the other hand, if he is unsympathetic to your feelings, chances are that he is addicted to his voyeurism and may suffer from other paraphilia as well.

- *He tries to look down a woman's blouse or up her skirt any time he can without being caught.* My first interaction with a patient who had voyeuristic tendencies was with a well-established businessman in his late forties who also suffered from premature ejaculation and erectile problems caused by excessive sexualized arousal. With great shame, he admitted that for many years he had surreptitiously glanced at a woman's cleavage at any opportunity. If, for example, a co-worker bent over and her blouse hung away from her breasts, he would try to "steal a peek." Occasionally he would even go slightly out of his way for a bit of tit. In detail he told me that if he were riding the subway and saw a woman with a low-cut top at the other end of the subway car, he would slowly maneuver himself closer and closer to her until he reached a viewing position.

I did not make much of his behavior until it became evident that it had somewhat of a compulsive quality. This was evidenced one day when as I was bending down to fill out his next appointment card, he said, "This is very hard for me to tell you, but I'm doing that looking thing right this moment." Had he not told me, I never would have known.

When we traced his history, what emerged was the picture of a young boy who did not begin dating until his early twenties because he felt physically unattractive. Over the course of his adolescence he had begun watching girls voyeuristically as a way of compensating for his feelings of powerlessness with women. He could look without their knowledge and without having to risk their rejection.

"Is this truly voyeurism?" you may be asking yourself. The answer is yes and no. There is no doubt that just like Peeping Tom, this man was violating the boundaries of the women he watched. They, like me, did not ask to be looked at. But this form of voyeurism is not an addiction because the behavior is not mandatory for arousal. In fact, the man I just discussed successfully overcame both his premature ejaculation and his erection problem. In addition, when I talked about this issue with a male colleague, he joked and said that he could imagine the whole subway carload of men trying to maneuver their way to see a great pair of boobs.

• *He frequents topless bars and peep shows.* Although harmless in itself, this behavior almost always is an indication of strong voyeuristic impulses. This kind of a man is addicted to the act of watching. What he does is take the turn-on from the peep show or bar and bring it into his fantasy life when he's having sex with his partner. You know he's an addict because when he tries to give up the peep shows and the fantasies, he usually begins having trouble with his erections.

This was the case with Patrick, a business executive in his mid-thirties. Out of guilt and a feeling that something was wrong, he tried weaning himself off going to the peeps as well as using fantasy with his wife. The less he fueled his fantasies, the more impotent he became. By the time he reached my office, Patrick was able to get an erection with his wife only fifty percent of the time.

- *He owns a pornography collection that would put most people in hock.* Watching pornographic films in itself would hardly raise an eyebrow in this day and age. In fact, many women are telling me that they, too, find watching erotic films exciting. However, there could be larger problems looming if a man spends an inordinate amount of time or money in the pursuit of pornography. If, for instance, you notice he has a pornography collection worth thousands of dollars, it is reasonable to suspect that he has a powerful voyeuristic tendency to which he is addicted. In all likelihood, he engages in Peeping Tom behavior as well. If you are not yet in a relationship with this man, it will be important for you to think about whether or not you want to become involved with someone who will need to undergo a great deal of treatment to overcome his addiction.

- *He owns sophisticated telescopic equipment, and you know he is not interested in astronomy.* At the more extreme end of the voyeur continuum there is the traditional Peeping Tom. Although his voyeurism may have begun as a child looking through windows, today's adult Peeping Tom has been completely transformed with advances in technology. Rather than look through peepholes, the male voyeur often has an array of expensive telescopic equipment that has been bought specifically for him covertly to watch others undress or engage in sexual activity. A man like this will spend time, energy, and often money planning as well as looking at those he selects. He is also powerless over his looking, even if the behavior costs him his reputation, relationship, or job.

A man like this is obviously an addict, and in all likelihood he engages in other addictive sexual behaviors. He needs professional help.

THE EXHIBITIONIST

It is normal for humans to display their bodies as part of courtship behavior. And there is a little bit of exhibitionism in the men who, for example, spend hours at the gym building up their bodies so that they can attract attention when they strut on the beach in their bikini swim trucks.

Exhibitionism of a pathological nature is a completely different animal. The purpose of the exhibitionist is not simply to get attention. He needs the element of surprise aimed at the recipient to produce his arousal.

My experience with exhibitionists suggests that the underlying cause of the behavior is an extreme feeling of inadequacy about masculinity. One twenty-seven-year-old man who described himself as a shy and gawky kid, whom girls teased and made fun of, began exposing himself at the age of ten as a way of showing off. "I remember feeling really proud of my erection. It symbolized that I was becoming a man. When I first began exposing myself to girls, it was not with the intention to frighten them but to show off."

Similar feelings of inadequacy were expressed by a young European man whom I will discuss in more detail below. He was the youngest of five brothers. His other brothers were tall and olive-skinned; he was fair. They all were men in his mother's eyes while he was still a boy. "The only way I didn't feel inadequate was in relationship to my penis," he told me. "I realized at a fairly young age that I was well endowed in this area." Of course, on a conscious level this man is well aware of the fact that exposing himself publicly is wrong. On an unconscious level, however, it is almost as if there were a little voice telling me, "If you have it, flaunt it."

How can you pinpoint a man who is an exhibitionist or has these tendencies? Except for exhibitionism in the most obvious form, this type of man is not always easy to detect.

- *He exposes himself inappropriately.* He is the guy who usually comes to mind when people think of an exhibitionist—the flasher in a trench coat. His arousal is completely contingent upon startling his victim. In fact, if you were calmly to ask such a man to put his penis back in his pants because it is not appropriate to expose oneself to the public, he would probably comply and his arousal would dissipate.

    Men who exhibit themselves regularly tend to be socially as well as sexually isolated. Some, however, are seemingly capable of engaging in what at first appears to be a normal sexual relationship. A man like this may flash either in public or in any other situation in which his victim is likely to be startled. In one unnerving incident that victim happened to be me. The man was in his mid-twenties, of European descent and handsome. His presenting problem was premature ejaculation. His exhibitionist tendencies quickly became clear, however. He began by telling me that he was proud of what he considered a larger-than-average penis, an asset that he told me he would like me to see. I defined clearly the parameters of our sessions and explicitly told him that this kind of acting out was not permissible. He held himself in check for a brief period. Then, one day, seemingly out of the clear blue, he entered a trancelike state. He proceeded to tell me that this was something that he had to do and began unzipping his pants. "I know I shouldn't do this, but I have to," he muttered. In a voice that was steady and firm, I told him that what he was doing was inappropriate, and I expected him to stop it. This maneuver broke him out of his trance.

    Uncomfortable with the possibility that this might recur, I referred him to a male psychiatrist.

- *He has a peculiar habit of leaving the window open when you make love.* Although he is unlikely to be direct about this at first, this type of exhibitionist will, within a short time in a new sexual relationship, make it a point to allow others to watch. You will know if a man like this has a serious problem by the insistent nature of his request. He will consistently express a very definitive preference for having sex in places that you can be seen and will become abusive when you resist these requests. Such a man has problems that run deep, and he should be avoided if you want a healthy sexual relationship.

SADOMASOCHISM

Men who are hooked into these activities, generally known as S and M, have issues of pain, dominance, and submission intertwined with their sexuality. Although no one knows for sure how these tendencies develop, it is believed that they originate from one of two places. The first is sexual guilt. Men who have come to experience great shame around their sexual feelings may be able to experience lust only after atoning for their guilty feelings about sex through self-inflicted or other-inflicted punishment.

It is also believed that the linkage between sex and pain can develop through an early association between corporal punishment and sexual arousal. More out of fear than actual pleasure, boys may get a panic erection when being spanked or whipped. As a result, there can develop a linkage between spanking and actual arousal.

Men with S and M tendencies run a wide gamut from enjoying light bondage to inflicting or receiving intense physical pain or verbal humiliation.

- *My partner enjoys sex only when I am the aggressor.* In all likelihood a man like this has grown up with a lot of negative messages about sex. He may believe that sex is forbidden as well as an intrusion on the woman he is with. As a result, he can enjoy sex only when the woman takes charge. If you initiate, he does not have to feel that he is somehow violating you. Also, if you do the initiating, he can imagine that you are "forcing" him to be sexual. This makes the forbidden more acceptable.

    A man called Gary comes to mind. Gary came to me complaining of erection problems, which amazingly seemed to disappear when he was with a sexually aggressive woman. His sexual fantasies typically involved light bondage. He would be tied to a bed, for example, and therefore unable to avoid the sexual advances of the woman in his fantasies. As I got to know Gary, the story that emerged was of a man whose father told him that sex would give him serious diseases and that unmarried women considered a sexual advance by a man nothing short of rape. These messages cost Gary a number of potentially successful relationships with women. Assuming that making a sexual advance would be viewed as an intrusion, Gary always waited for the woman he was courting to make the first move. Unfortunately, since ours is a society in which it is still expected that the male be the sexual aggressor, the women on the receiving end interpreted Gary's behavior to mean that he was either not interested or gay. In a few instances when a woman broke out of the traditional mold and initiated a sexual relationship, Gary was able to enjoy the sexual contact so long as she took the sexual lead. In essence, this meant that he would touch his partner genitally only if she did so first or would have intercourse only if she initiated it. Over time the few women he was with sexually began to resent his passivity and terminated the relationships.

If you are in a relationship like this, the chances of the man's resolving this problem with therapy are excellent. What he needs to do, as Gary did, is to understand the origins of his negative messages about sex as well as to learn, with the partner's help, that sex is healthy and fun and that women enjoy it.

• *My partner has expressed an interest in sex games that involve light bondage.* The fantasy of being "raped"—that is, being forced to submit to a woman's sexual whims and desires—is widespread among men. It may be that your partner's expression of interest is little more than a desire to act out playfully something he has dreamed about for years. Again, if you feel okay about participating, there is no harm done. Nor is this necessarily an indication that there is a deeper problem working beneath the surface, particularly if such a game is played with limited frequency and is not a condition for your partner's sexual pleasure.

If, on the other hand, it becomes clear that he *needs* to incorporate bondage games into your sex life on a regular basis, chances are that he is, or has the potential to become, addicted to this kind of behavior for arousal. This is really what separates pathological from nonpathological S and M behavior. There are many men (and women) who seem to enjoy what are often called "playful" S and M games. These games can include everything from light bondage to light humiliation to mild spanking, which are not particularly painful. But these same individuals also enjoy and function perfectly well with only "straight" sex. Nor do they need to escalate the severity of the "punishment" to keep the S and M games interesting.

Still, the line between "playful" S and M and abusive masochistic behavior is arbitrary and has a lot to do with what our society considers acceptable.

- *He enjoys it when I command him to perform sexual acts.*

or

- *He is aroused when he is spanked or whipped or otherwise hurt physically.* Although the behaviors are highly variable in terms of content and degree, a man chronically exhibiting any of the above needs the element of punishment before he allows himself to take pleasure in what he perceives as "sinful" lust. Many people wonder how anyone can become aroused by being humiliated or how pain can be any sort of turn-on. The answer is that often the S and M addict is not. What is really going on here is that being humiliated or hurt provides the sufficient psychological condition of having paid for the man's sexual feelings and clears a pathway for his becoming aroused.

Unlike men who are into playful S and M, a man who enjoys being abused or being abusive sexually almost always suffers from not only a serious sexual dysfunction but an emotional one as well. As a result, he becomes terribly isolated socially. Furthermore, he is so ashamed of his sexual behavior and fantasies that he becomes even more isolated. A man with these S and M tendencies is a poor choice if you are looking for a healthy partner, because he has a fundamental inability to love both himself and others.

Lester is such a man. Despite his good looks, he had had only one emotional and sexual involvement with a woman in his life. Sadly that ended in disaster because she did not share his interest in sadomasochistic behavior. Lester's need to be punished came out in both fantasy and actuality. His most frequent fantasy was of being the bull in a bullfighting ring where all the matadors were females with spiked heels. Rather than use daggers, they would kick and step on him with their sharp heels. When he would begin to bleed, he would have an orgasm.

Lester's pattern of arousal in actuality was similar. He made frequent visits to numerous dominatrices. He would be their slave, and they would command him to lick their shoes and feet. They would then tell him that he had not done this adequately and therefore needed a kicking and spanking. As he was being beaten and humiliated, his arousal would peak.

What emerged in our sessions together was the painful story of unrequited boyish love for his mother. Lester recalled believing at a very young age that his mother was the most beautiful woman in the world. His feelings became eroticized somehow when Lester, who was about six years old at the time, found a pair of his mother's hose and experienced a sexual kind of rush from smelling them. Lester's mother was oblivious not only of these feelings but of Lester. Cold and withdrawn, she did not hide the fact that Lester's older brother, Steven, was her favorite. As she increasingly put him down, two things happened. His erotic feelings toward her began to intensify in the form of the fantasy that became a staple in his sexual arousal. Ridden with shame and guilt about his sexual feelings as well as the humiliation of his mother's rejection, he increasingly turned inward. Over many years Lester developed a world into which no one else was allowed to enter in any truly intimate way.

As is the case with many individuals who suffer from a serious sexual addiction, Lester was unable to stick it out in treatment. Despite the fact that he began attending Sexual Compulsives Anonymous meetings, he was unable to stop acting out. To do so would have forced him to confront his terrible loneliness and fear of being rejected. That is why as soon as Lester realized that he was beginning to let me in and to feel a connection with me, he became terribly frightened and fled.

The pain of the Lesters of the world is profound. However, if you know such a man, you would be misleading yourself as well as him if you thought that you alone had the ability to turn him around. Some sex addicts, if they spend years in treatment, are able to recover. Sadly, most have difficulty committing themselves to any relationship, including a therapeutic one. That is why the prognosis for such a man is poor.

COERCIVE SEX

Coercive sex refers to verbally or physically forcing sex on someone else. The most obvious example is stranger rape, a crime of power rather than passion. Men who are rapists or sexual predators of this kind can experience lust only when there is a lack of consent from their partners. Obviously a man with this type of history is pathologically disturbed.

But there are other forms of intrusive or inappropriate sex that are much more subtle and insidious, leaving the person on the receiving end feeling violated although she is often unsure why. A man exhibiting these behaviors is almost always sexually insecure and gains a feeling of being in control by making his "victim" feel uncomfortable.

- *He always seems to bring up the subject of sex or jokes about sex even when it seems inappropriate.* This is by far the most familiar form of coercive sex, and it can occur in almost any situation. You may notice, for example, that a man you know frequently seems to bring up the subject of sex, often out of the blue. Always it seems inappropriate, although at times it is difficult to pinpoint why.

  One woman's experience with a psychotherapist is a case in point. Although the therapist never made any direct advances toward her and she never felt unsafe with him in that way, she told me that eventually she began noticing that he made a comment of a sexual nature in virtually every session. For example, she asked him how often he thought she should come, meaning how often she should come in for treatment. "I think you should come in here once a week," he told her, "but a good come, more often than not, is always good for the body and mind." On another occasion, she was discussing the issue of ethics and ambition. She was describing someone in her office who seemed overly concerned with morality because she turned down a promotion since she knew that an older gentleman in the office whose wife was dying of cancer needed the money more.

"I am not heartless, but I never would have done that," she told the therapist.

"You would have given the boss a blow job if you needed to," he responded.

As obvious as his sexual remarks might seem, two things clouded the issue for this woman. First, the therapist was genuinely helping her. Second, a number of these remarks were made when both she and her husband were seeing this therapist for couples counseling. "The truth is, if my husband hadn't been there on a number of these occasions, I would have begun to wonder if I was provoking him in some way," she told me.

Whether coming from a stranger, friend, or therapist, this type of verbal behavior is an intrusion. What the man behind the behavior is truly about, though, can be difficult to know for certain. Some men are uncomfortable about sex and their sexuality and use this tactic as a way of covering up their vulnerability. The men that come into my office with vocabularies that are limited to four-letter words are good examples. For other men, talking in this provocative way may be a power play, with the intention of making you feel uncomfortable and diminished. There is also the possibility that a man like this is simply crude: that he is a dirty old man, regardless of his age. In this case he may be completely oblivious of just how offensive or, in some cases, just how ridiculous he appears.

• *When he touches you, there is always something covertly sexual about it.* Although intrusive, lot of things might be going on here. He may be interested in having an affair with you, and this is his way of letting you know. Then, of course, there is always a good possibility that he has PE and therefore knows no other way to touch. If he is potentially an addict, he is getting off by touching you in this sexual way and using that arousal to fuel his fantasies later on.

Whatever the cause, if you are uncomfortable with this sort of touching, the best way to stop it is to confront directly the person doing it. If the behavior stops from that point on, you have not been dealing with anything too serious. If, on the other hand, it continues or, even worse, seems to become exaggerated, there is a good likelihood that this man's sexuality is very much linked to coercion and power. Just how far he will go to become aroused through coercive means is unknown. If you know a man like this, proceed with caution.

• *He asks you to dress seductively so that he can show you off to other men.* Being with a sexy, attractive woman is a boost to most men's egos. And there is a type of man who tries to get his partner to change her hairdo or dress in a certain way to fit the image of what he would like her to be. A man like this is usually unhappy with his partner and tries to change her exterior in hopes that his feelings about her will change. But he should not be confused with a man who needs his partner to dress in a particular way in order for him to become aroused.

The paraphiliac who insists that his partner dress in a blatantly sexual way does so for the express purpose of getting other men to look at and respond to her. He does not care whether or not his partner feels comfortable dressing in this way. That is because the objectification of his partner is often a crucial component to his arousal. A man like this often loves his partner. At the same time he usually has a lot of guilt about sex and sexual feelings. His way of circumventing those feelings is to turn his partner into an object of other men's fantasies. He then can use this imagery to help override his own shame and discomfort about sex.

It is the coercive nature of this man's needs that makes him a problem. There are a lot of women who enjoy dressing up in a sexy way and playfully showing off their wares, to the delight of both other men and the women's partners. This is harmless. But if your partner insists that you dress or act in a certain way despite the fact that it makes you feel uncomfortable, you have a serious problem that almost always requires professional intervention to resolve.

• *He insists on or tries to push you into having sex with another man or woman in his presence.* He is usually a more seriously disturbed version of the man discussed above. This person can become aroused only if a person he loves is defiled in some way.

Gregory is a good example. He and his fiancée, Nancy, had a lusty sex life before they were married. Reared as a staunch Catholic, Gregory had internalized the idea that sex before marriage was forbidden; this made Nancy a sinner in their premarital days. This all changed when the wedding bells chimed. In the course of a few months Gregory found it almost impossible to sustain an erection. Under the ruse of telling Nancy that he felt that he had missed out on a lot sexually and wanted to be sexually experimental with her, Gregory set up a series of threesomes. Some involved men, and others women. At first Nancy found these experiences titillating. But after a while she began to feel exploited. "I just wanted to have normal sex with my husband," she told me in tears. "But the only time he seemed to be able to be turned on was during or shortly after a sexual experience with other people involved." This response is typical for a sex addict of this type. And it will not change on its own. Gregory is presently in long-term one-to-one treatment and is attending Sexual Compulsives Anonymous groups in order to overcome his addiction. So should any man who experiences such a problem.

• *You wake up in the middle of the night and discover your partner having intercourse with you.* This may or may not suggest an intrusive tendency. For example, this behavior is not rare among men who suffer from chronic erection problems. Many have told me that if they wake up with erections, they feel driven to try to use them. Some sex therapists actually suggest that a man with a serious erection dysfunction try this technique. They think that when his partner is asleep and therefore undemanding, his performance anxiety might be reduced sufficiently to let him have successful intercourse.

Sometimes a man may simply wake up feeling horny. Since most men would not mind if their partners initiated sex while they were asleep, he may assume that she would not mind either. In fact, some women do not mind and enjoy this impromptu advance.

If, on the other hand, you do feel offended, and your partner still refuses to stop, he is engaging in wife rape.

- *He wakes you up in the middle of the night even though you've told him many times that you don't enjoy it.*

or

- *When you tell him that you're not in the mood, he verbally badgers you until you finally just give in.*

or

- *He tries to coerce you into performing certain sexual acts that you don't feel comfortable with.* If you think that intrusive sex occurs only between nonintimates, think again. Wife rape, or engaging in sex with a partner without mutual consent, is much more common than a lot of people think. At the extreme there is a small minority of men who become physically violent when their wives don't put out for them sexually. But most forms of wife rape involve verbal and emotional rather than physical battering.

What kind of man is prone to this type of coercion? Almost always it is someone who, on some level, views his wife as a kind of possession. Regarding a wife as someone to service him, he does not think that her permission or consent is required or even necessary for him to have sex with her. Invariably this attitude of a wife's being a kind of possession comes out in the way he relates to her generally.

Also, a man like this often has other emotional problems, such as manic depression. Even if he doesn't, there is little doubt that this sort of guy is incapable of true intimacy.

Interestingly, a number of women I have spoken to do not openly complain to their partners when this happens despite the fact that they feel violated. In some cases the women may be afraid that their partners will react by becoming physically violent. In other instances women have been taught to be submissive, particularly concerning their spouses. A woman, like her husband, might consider herself to be her husband's property. Then there are women who were sexually abused as children and have come to expect that they will be taken advance of sexually and that there is nothing they can do to stop it.

Some women, of course, do speak up. Occasionally the problem is simply a lack of communication. Your partner cannot know that you do not enjoy what you are doing unless you tell him. Even if it is obvious that you are not totally into it, he may interpret your lack of direct communication to mean that you feel neutral about the subject. You may not like it, but neither do you dislike it.

If you do speak up and still find yourself ignored, you should seek professional help. You are in an abusive relationship and need to find the way out.

THE MALE NYMPHOMANIAC

Although there is little doubt that women are capable of enjoying sex a great deal, there seems to be some truth to the idea that men are more sexually motivated than women. "All he thinks about is sex" is not an uncommon complaint among women. When women become stressed, from either work or children, their sex drive often goes down the tubes. This is not equally true for a man. On the contrary, sex may be a good way for a man to alleviate stress.

This male/female discrepancy in drive should not be confused with a man whose sex drive has gone awry.

- *His need for sexual relief has an addictive quality.* You may get the feeling, for example, that he just doesn't *want* to have sex with you but *needs* to have sex. This may become apparent when you notice that he regularly shuns other responsibilities in order to have his sexual needs met. You also are likely to notice that whenever you speak to him, he talks obsessively about sex or plans future sexual contact.

- *He masturbates compulsively.* A lot of pubescent boys masturbate three or four times a day for a period of time. The sexually compulsive male can masturbate even more often than that. In fact, he may overstimulate himself to the point of hurting his genitals.
- *He says he loves me and behaves lovingly toward me, but he cannot seem to stop having sex with other women.* There are a number of possibilities here. He may simply have a fear of intimacy and therefore be unwilling to make a commitment. Or perhaps he has the kind of desire disorder that makes it difficult for him to feel comfortable with having sex with someone he loves.

The sex addict's problems go much deeper. For a man like this, sex is a fix, and he will go to almost any length and take almost any risk to have it. He suffers from the Madonna–whore conflict mentioned earlier, but to an extreme. For a male nymphomaniac, there is a gap between love and lust. He has replaced his desperate need for love with lust, although he often does not consciously know it. And because he feels so deprived and unsure that anyone could truly love him, he needs to be with a different partner with compulsive frequency.

A good example is Ted, a thirty-two-year-old disc jockey for a major radio station. Ted had been in an eight-year relationship with a woman named Blaire whom he professed to love very much. His infidelities had broken up the relationship numerous times. Each time Ted went back to Blaire, begging for her forgiveness, and swore he would give up his sexual escapades. His commitment when he made it was in earnest. The problem is that like any addict, he was out of control over his addiction.

Ted, who lives in another state, came to me for help when Blaire gave him an ultimatum: that he either resolve his problem or forgo the relationship. I told Ted that he would need to attend Sexual Compulsives Anonymous meetings as part of his recovery, a suggestion he rejected. Just like many addicts, he was convinced he could resolve the problem without going public. It became clear, even to Ted, that he was out of control when four months into his treatment he came to his appointment with me forty minutes late. The reason was that he had been picked up by a call girl on the street and felt unable to resist her. It was also evident that Ted was unwilling to make the tremendous commitment it takes to overcome a sexual addiction. That was our last session.

Ted is very typical of such a sex addict. He has multiple and often anonymous partners and has no respect for risk. In addition, he will pay for sex, even if it means depleting his financial resources. If you have just met up with such a man, you'd be wise to look elsewhere for a relationship.

ADDICTS AND PARAPHILIACS:
A PROGNOSIS

Unless you are already committed to a relationship with a partner who suffers from a paraphilia or an addiction, it is probably best to disengage. The prognosis for these individuals is iffy at best. Even when there is a successful outcome, treatment is almost always a lengthy and difficult process.

There are a number of treatment options available for men with these problems although usually therapy involves a combination of interventions. There are certain drugs, such as Depo-Provera, that seem to relieve sexual tension and agitation. These antiandrogenic drugs seem to have the effect of reducing the drive of the sexual compulsive. Long-term individual treatment combined with regular self-help meetings can also be beneficial, particularly for the man who is not in a committed relationship.

Resolving the problems of the paraphiliac who has a steady partner is another ball game entirely. That is because most women who are involved over long periods with sex addicts or paraphiliacs are part of the problem.

There are two types of woman who hook up with this sort of guy. Frequently she herself is someone who suffers from a paraphilia or a sexual addiction. Not surprisingly, that addiction often matches the one of her partner or at least can be made to match reasonably well. The result is two people who are mutually engaged in their addictions. Unless those addictions are dangerous or of a criminal nature, these individuals rarely hit rock bottom and can live a lifetime acting out sexually.

Then there is the type of woman who is completely oblivious of her partner's secret sexual life. Sometimes everyone in the world knows of his problem but she. Other times she may ignore a bulk of facts that don't fit together. If you suspect that you might be this woman, then it is important for you to recognize that you have your own serious issues that attract you to a sex addict to begin with, and that keep you in denial about his addiction. And unless you are committed to helping yourself, you are involved in keeping the problem alive.

PART TWO

WHAT
YOU
CAN DO

7

Conditions for Change

"I love Bruce and want to marry him," Janice, an attractive twenty-eight-year-old paralegal, told me. Her head was bowed as if she were embarrassed to look either me or her fiancé squarely in the eye. "And I don't want to make Bruce feel our relationship is on the line because of his coming too fast because I know that will only put more pressure on him, and the last thing I want to do is to make the problem worse. But," she said, lowering her voice further, "the truth is that it does bother me." Then, as if apologizing, she turned to Bruce. "I can't help it. It makes sex less enjoyable for me. I love you and want to be with you. But it is very important that we work on this together."

It's obvious that it is excruciatingly painful for a man to have a sexual problem. But it is also terribly hurtful for the woman who lives with that man. And it can be extremely frustrating not to know what to do about the problem.

In this chapter you will learn the prerequisites for overcoming the problem and the steps you can take to begin resolving it.

CONDITIONS FOR CHANGE

Four fundamental prerequisites need to be met before you can begin to address the problem. First, you need a problem that is not so deeply rooted that it cannot be resolved with sex therapy techniques. Some difficulties are so profound that a man may have to go through a course of psychotherapy before the approaches in this book will have any impact.

Second, you need to be a woman who is in a position sexually to help him change. In most cases, this means that you yourself need to be relatively free of sexual conflicts and inhibitions. If you are conflicted about sex, you may have an unconscious motivation to keep your partner dysfunctional as a way to avoid facing your own inhibitions. In fact, your problem may be exacerbating your partner's problem.

Third, you need to have a good feeling about your partner and the relationship. Working with a man to overcome a sexual problem requires love, patience, and understanding, and if you are seething with unresolved hostility, it will be impossible for you to be in a therapeutic state of mind.

Finally, you need a man who recognizes that he has a problem and is motivated to change it. You also need a man who is motivated to change it with *you*.

In some instances you and your partner may be able to work through the problem without professional intervention. In other instances you will need the assistance of a certified sex therapist to overcome the difficulty. Either way, it is important that you recognize that sexual problems are laden with enormous emotional overtones for both people in the relationship. And while the rewards of working through a sexual problem can be enormous, in terms not only of your sex life but of the general level of intimacy, getting there may require traveling through some rocky territory.

PREREQUISITE 1: HE HAS A PROBLEM
YOU CAN HELP HIM SOLVE

Pamela was a sexually dysfunctional man's dream woman. A registered nurse, she had all the patience and positive nurturing instincts that facilitate healing. She also had taken courses on her own in human sexuality so she was an informed partner . . . or so she believed. When

Pamela met Fred, a man in his early thirties who confessed that he suffered from a chronic impotence problem, she made it her mission to help him get over his erection difficulties. Given her knowledge about impotence and the performance anxiety that is often at the root of the problem, Pamela told Fred that he should simply forget about intercourse until he felt ready. She showed him other ways of pleasuring her and paid a lot of attention to Fred's genitals during foreplay until she saw he was becoming anxious, at which point she focused on other parts of his body. She never complained and was endlessly hopeful that once Fred relaxed, he would be able to achieve penetration. She even got a colleague to give her some Viagra for Fred to try.

Her patience was to no avail. After six months Fred had achieved penetration only once, and even then he had been able to stay hard inside her for just a brief time. By now Pamela was becoming frustrated and suggested Fred come in for a consultation with me. A preliminary history revealed the possibility of sexual abuse, although Fred did not remember this at the time. I spent several sessions tracing Fred's childhood, and within a few months he was having powerful flashbacks of having been molested by his uncle. It became apparent that Fred's erection problem was only a symptom of the more profound problems related to the abuse. It was those problems that needed to be resolved before sex therapy could have any chance of success. Pamela was not wrong for wanting to help. She simply did not know, or did not want to believe, that Fred's problem was too serious for her to handle on her own. Pamela could have tried every exercise in this book, could have had endless patience, and she would have had no success.

How, then, can you avoid this kind of frustration? What is the best way to assess whether your partner's sexual problem is amenable to the treatment exercises in this book? Below are some guidelines that will help you make that determination. While there are no hard-and-fast rules, it is generally true that the more conscious the cause, the more easily resolvable the problem.

Premature ejaculation: This is almost always resolvable, but getting good results is likely to be more difficult and take a longer period of time if:

- He is extremely anxious about the problem.
- He is sexually immature or inexperienced.
- He is uncomfortable about masturbation.
- He comes from a very religious background.
- There are other difficulties present, such as an erection problem or general sexual inexperience.

Erection problems: These are almost always resolvable, except under the following circumstances:

- He has a long-term history of erection problems, with short periods of remission. This usually suggests a psychological problem that first needs to be resolved. If you are in a new relationship and the problem does not get better once you are more comfortable with each other, chances are good that there is a deeper problem at work.
- He has not really have an erection problem but, rather, a desire problem related to his feelings about you. (You will not know this unless he tells you he's had an affair and is fully functional in that context.)
- The problem has a large organic component. Here medical intervention may be necessary. However, since most erection problems, even those physically based, have a psychological component, combining medical intervention with the suggested exercises presented in this section can be beneficial.

A combination of an erection problem and premature ejaculation: This is almost always resolvable (except if either is caused by the conditions noted just above), although the erection problem needs to be dealt with first.

Low sexual desire: If the problem is related to you or your relationship, it is resolvable if the issues causing it can be resolved first. If the problem stems from deeper origins, such as conflicts about love and intimacy, the help of a therapist to work through these issues is almost always necessary.

Simple sexual inexperience: This can be relatively easy to resolve if the man has simply missed this stage of development and has a patient partner.

Sexual inexperience caused by conflicts about women or about gender preference: Usually professional help is necessary because of the deep-rooted psychological aspect of this problem. You may be able to help a man overcome the sexual problem but be left with someone who abandons the relationship because of his conflicts about intimacy with women. However, a combination of professional help and the exercises in this book can be effective, even among men who begin with strong conflicts about sex.

Sexual aversions and inhibited male orgasm: Although these can be resolved they are difficult problems to overcome. If, as is generally the case, the struggle to climax is combined with inexperience and conflict or ambivalence about intimacy, professional intervention is usually necessary.

Paraphilias: These are extremely difficult to resolve, with or without professional help. A man with a paraphilia might learn to be able to respond to women in a more normal fashion, but his need for the paraphilia is usually an addiction that is difficult to erase.

Any problem caused by sexual abuse should always be treated professionally to avoid triggering recollections of the original abuse that you may not be able to deal with effectively.

PREREQUISITE 2: YOU ARE FREE OF SEXUAL PROBLEMS

Once you have determined that your partner has a solvable problem, the next step is to figure out whether or not you are in a position to help him. A woman with her own unresolved sexual issues needs to deal with and to work through those issues before she can work with a sexually dysfunctional partner. That's because a woman's sexual problems can wreak havoc on the sexual equilibrium of a relationship.

Nicole and Matthew's relationship is a good example. When I first met Nicole, she was a walking volcano because of the negative effect that Matthew's premature ejaculations were having on their sexual relationship. Matthew did have a moderate problem with premature ejaculation; by his own description, he was rarely able to last more than three or four minutes after penetration. The angrier Nicole became with him, the more pressure she put on him, the worse his problem became. Upon closer scrutiny, however, it became clear that Nicole's complaints about Matthew were a way of taking the heat off her own problem with having orgasms. Here was Nicole bitching about Matthew's inability to last with penetration, yet she had never had an orgasm during intercourse even though she had been with several very healthy partners before she was married, none of whom had control problems. In fact, Matthew was the only man with whom she had ever had an orgasm. When she did have an orgasm, it occurred only after twenty-five minutes of very intense manual stimulation. As long as Nicole could point her finger at Matthew and his problem, she could avoid looking at her own.

I am not blaming women for men's sexual problems. If, however, you are sexually dysfunctional or inhibited, it may be very difficult for you to help a partner work through his problems. A woman who is sexually ill at ease tends to exaggerate, contribute to, or, in some instances, be the primary cause of her partner's problems.

If you rarely or never have orgasms with a partner, or do not have much interest in sex, or are inhibited about sexual intimacy, these difficulties are likely to affect your ability to help your partner in numerous ways:

- *You will not be very interested in sex and will tend to cut the experience short.* I do not care what you may tell yourself, the fact is that unless you have orgasms, you do not enjoy sex very much. Women who say that orgasms do not matter are not in touch with their sexuality. I do not mean that if on occasion you fail to climax, you do not have a satisfying sex life. And once in a while it may suffice just to feel emotionally close to your partner through sex. I also do not mean to suggest that you have to be orgasmic with intercourse alone. Many women who enjoy sex have orgasms easily from manual stimulation, but are unable to climax regularly simply from the thrusting of the penis in the vagina. But if you do not reach orgasm regularly in one way or another, your enjoyment of and interest in sex will not be very high.

If you do not have orgasms or are inhibited about sex, you will not have a great deal of internal motivation to prolong your sexual experiences. If your partner has premature ejaculation, it will be boring at best and uncomfortable at worst for you to slow down the pace of foreplay, which is a necessary component of resolving that problem. In addition, if you do not have orgasms at all or think that you are unable to come with penetration, you may thrust quickly and make your partner come fast in order to get it over with.

If your partner is experiencing impotence or a desire disorder, your impulse to rush through lovemaking will make life difficult for him. If you are trying to rush things, you may not give your partner the type of stimulation he needs in order to achieve and sustain an erection. If you touch his genitals in a mechanical way, he is likely to have trouble responding. Finally, if he picks up the message that you want to finish, you increase his performance pressure, which ultimately only makes his difficulties worse.

As a result, it will be hard for you to sustain the kind of motivation necessary to help your partner overcome his problem. Emotionally you may very much want to be there for him and alleviate his suffering and embarrassment. At the same time you have a built-in motivation to avoid sexual activity because sex is not all that pleasurable for you. Time and again I have seen a woman who is nonorgasmic zealously jump into the exercises to help her partner, only to lose interest over time. As one woman, who finally realized that she had to deal with her orgasm problem before she could help her husband with his erection problem, put it, "My heart was willing. But it became very difficult for me to show the kind of interest in sex I know he wanted me to have because there was no physical reward in it for me."

Unless you are generally interested in sex and find it pleasing, your motivation will be very limited, and eventually inertia is likely to set in.

- *Your partner may be less likely to want to work on his problem with you because he will think that it makes little difference to you.* As one husband told me, "Why should I knock myself out trying to last longer during intercourse when I know my wife will not derive any more pleasure than she does now?"

What do you do if you have seen yourself in the past few pages? How do you proceed if you acknowledge that your partner is not the only one in your relationship with a sexual problem? I suggest you set up an appointment with a sex therapist and begin working on your own problem first. The American Association of Sex Educators, Counselors and Therapists, in Chicago, will be happy to provide you with a list of qualified therapists in your area. After you resolve your own conflicts, your partner's problem can take on a very different perspective.

Also, owning up to your contribution to the problem often paves the way for a man to be more amenable to taking responsibility for his problem. Men are generally resistant to therapy to begin with and are more defensive when they are dragged into treatment because of a problem women define as *their* problem. However, if you are able to tell your partner that you need his help working on the problem, this can be a door opener for examining and working on the whole of your sexual relationship in a less threatening way. This is a good approach for every woman who wants to encourage her partner's involvement. It is essential for a woman who has sexual problems herself.

PREREQUISITE 3: AN EMOTIONAL
READINESS TO HELP

The third ingredient necessary for successful working through a sexual problem is the ability to act therapeutically. It takes a great deal of commitment, coupled with the right frame of mind, to help a man resolve a sexual problem. Not only do you need to be a loving partner, but you need to act like, and in many ways adopt the role of, "therapist" to your partner as you practice the exercises in the following chapters. You need to have what I call a therapeutic mind-set.

There are several dimensions of this state of mind:

- *You need to have a good feeling about your relationship and your partner.* Whether your relationship is two weeks or twenty years old, if you do not have a fundamentally positive feeling about your partner, if there is too much unresolved anger, if you want to fight rather than heal, it will be impossible to work on the problem. In fact, in a tension-laden relationship, you may even have an unconscious stake in keeping the problem alive.

   If the relationship is in trouble for nonsexual reasons, you need to resolve those problems first. It takes a lot of goodwill and compassion to help a man whose ego is bruised to carry out successfully the treatment program presented in the following chapters.

- *You cannot judge your partner negatively for having a sexual problem.* This may seem obvious, but a lot of women, even those who feel generally good about the men they are with, often experience a type of reverse sexism that suggests that their partners are less of a man if they have sexual problems. We, as women, have been subjected to the same social imprinting that says that a man is not supposed to be weak and have prob- lems—period—let alone sexual difficulties. "I adore Tom, but the fact that he has these things [premature ejaculation and some erectile difficulty] makes me think less of him as a man somehow" is the way a thirty-two-year-old mother of two put it. "I know that's a terrible thing to say, especially since he is really a great husband and father. But I just can't help feeling that there is something wrong with him because he has these problems."

   Although she is far from alone, this kind of attitude is

obviously troublesome. You cannot work with a man on a sexual problem with a positive outlook if deep down you think he is fundamentally flawed.

It helps, first and foremost, to separate the problem from the man, to think of him as a man with a problem rather than as a sexually inadequate man. You also need to take a hard look at your sexist biases and begin accepting how unfair they are. To the extent that you give credence to the myth that men should always be more sexually expert, interested, and adept than women, you are more a part of the problem than of the cure.

- *You must be temporarily willing to put your own sexual needs aside.* While you are working on the exercises to help with your partner's problem, it will be crucial that you understand you are there to help *him.* There may be times when working on the problem will be sexually pleasurable for you, but there will also be times that in order to help him, you may need to have sexual contact when you are not particularly in the mood.

- *You must be patient.* Even if his problem is not very serious or complicated, change takes time. If you insist on a quick fix, your own impatience or uncertainty can contribute to your partner's already skyrocketing performance anxiety. But focusing on the overall path rather than on each step along the way can go a long way in helping alleviate your impatience. Things will *not* get better each and every time you work on the problem. On the contrary, there will be occasions when it seems as if you are making no progress or even backtracking. That does not mean that his problem is getting worse. As long as the general direction is positive, things are going well. If you have faith in the future of your relationship, it makes it easier to "keep your eye on the prize" as you go through the ups and downs of overcoming the problem. This does not mean that you will never feel upset, that you never get frustrated, or that you need to be perfect. It does mean that you have to be persistent, relax, and enjoy the process.

PREREQUISITE 4: A WILLING PARTNER

You may be ready and willing to help, and he may definitely have a problem, but without a man who wants to be helped, you will be fighting a losing battle.

Consider Hal, a famous entertainment maven in his mid-sixties who came to see me after what he described as a yearlong harangue by his wife. Hal told me that he had lost all sexual desire—period. He told me that he had never really been amorous, even in his younger years. Now he had no desire to masturbate or have sex with his wife or anyone else. His libido had come to a virtual standstill.

"Maybe I have a problem like my wife says," he admitted, shrugging his shoulders. "But I am not interested in solving it. I mean, it's hard to have interest when you don't feel desire, and never had much to begin with. The truth is, I am here only because of my wife. Actually," he added with a twisted smile, "I'm here just so I can get her off my back. So, do you think you can help me?"

"Only if you want to be helped," I responded.

"Well, I guess I really don't care," he answered cordially.

"Then I can't help you," I answered honestly.

"Well," he said, "at least I can tell my wife I spoke to somebody. Maybe that will calm her down."

"I doubt it," I thought. Still, unless a man wants to work on his problem, there is nothing that anyone can do to help him. Even if your partner wants to solve his problem, you will have a lion's share of resistance to overcome since he is bound to find some of the exercises threatening or difficult from what he believes will help him. Without his desire to solve the problem at the outset, there will be many hurdles, probably too many to make working on the problem worthwhile. The success rate is not very high for couples when the man is dragged in, kicking and screaming, by his wife.

At this point you may be wondering, "Why *wouldn't* a man want to work to overcome his problem?" There are many possibilities.

- *He does not care.* Up to this point the emphasis in this book has been on the pain and embarrassment most men with sexual problems experience. But not all men feel that way. There are some men, fortunately a minority, who are selfish, sexually and otherwise, and have no desire to change themselves in any way. Most typical of this charming sort of gentleman is the premature ejaculator who is every bit the "wham-bam-thank-you-ma'am" SOB who gives PE its bad reputation.

Then there are men like Hal who have lost sexual desire and do not care about regaining it. Or a man with health problems may believe that the inability to get an erection is the least of his problems. And of course, there is the man who has come not to care because his long-term partner seems not to care.

- *He does not think he has a problem.* It is very difficult to feel motivated to work on a problem when you believe that your functioning is perfectly adequate. And a surprising number of men who have problems honestly believe they are perfectly fine. Irving, for instance, was a fifty-four-year-old store owner who begrudgingly agreed to come see me with his second wife. Rose, to whom he had been married for two years. Rose bitterly complained that Irving had a serious premature ejaculation problem. Although Irving acknowledged that he did not have voluntary control over his orgasms, he refuted the idea of having a problem with the argument that he usually did last three or four minutes after penetration. "I read that the average American male lasts two and a half minutes," he said, citing an old Kinsey statistic. "So that makes me at least a little better than average. More to the point," he added, "my former wife never once complained, and neither did the other women I was with before and between marriages." Indeed, it took a good deal of convincing for Irving to accept the fact that a lot of women are loath to bring up a man's sexual problem for fear of injuring his ego and that this does not mean that a problem does not exist.

Another type of man who is hard to convince is one who was reared in a macho environment. Typically he's not into kissing, doesn't spend a lot of time on foreplay, thinks sensuality is stupid, and likes to get right to intercourse. In essence a man like this has a PE lovemaking style, except he doesn't have PE. Men like this tend to have grown up belonging to tough or pseudo-tough peer groups whose primary sexual motivation was to "score" and whose women were more or less sexual objects.

Another reason that a man with a problem may not take his problem seriously is that he believes his difficulty is temporary and will disappear by itself. Jim, a man in his late forties who eventually did come for help for his erection problem, had a year earlier refused to go for treatment despite his wife's prodding. The fact that his penis was not working was obvious. But he had also been under excruciating job stress, struggling to keep his company from filing for bankruptcy for eighteen months. Jim believed that his erection problems were a direct result of those external pressures; when the stress lifted, so would his penis.

If you are in a situation where your partner is convinced that something external is causing the trouble, you may have to wait it out before you can prove his theory wrong and gain his cooperation.

• *He knows he has a problem, but he's not committed enough to your relationship to work on it with you.* If you are in a new relationship, for example, the man you are with may recognize he has a problem but simply may not care or feel intimate enough to work on it with you. There is a lot of vulnerability that a man must confront if he is to resolve any sexual problem. If your present partner does not see a long-term future with you, he may not want to risk that exposure.

Often, too, a man may choose not to work on his problem with a woman he does not intend to have a long-term relationship with because he may feel he is using her. One sexually inexperienced patient was dating a woman he liked, but he knew in his heart of hearts that he didn't want to make a long-term commitment to her. He spoke for countless others when he said, "How could I ask her to help me solve this in good conscience? Even if I were totally up front with my feelings about the relationship, I would still feel that if she spent this time working with me on this, I would owe her something I don't want to owe."

A man in a long-term relationship may also not want to work on the problem if he is unhappy or wants out of the relationship. Then, of course, there is the possibility that it only looks as if he has a problem but that in reality he has a problem functioning only with you.

• *He senses that his sexual problem is symptomatic of a deeper problem in the relationship and is afraid of confronting it.* Years ago I worked with a delightful man in his fifties who was suffering from an increasingly recalcitrant case of impotence. For a year or so he did little, save wish and hope to resolve the problem. He never asked his partner to give him the genital stimulation he suspected he needed to function. Without speaking to her about the problem, this rather shy and up until now monogamous man had a few brief affairs to reaffirm his potency. He discovered his hunch was correct: When he was with a woman who spent time touching him before intercourse, his erections were no problem at all.

The solution to resolving his problem with his wife seemed obvious. All he needed to do was to let her know about his need for more direct stimulation of his penis. Yet for weeks he resisted communicating this information to her. It did not take long before it became apparent that something was holding him back. That something, it turned out, was a paralyzing fear that his wife had fallen out of love with him, that their sexual problems were only the tip of the iceberg. He was absolutely terrified that if they began addressing the sexual issue, he would be opening a Pandora's box.

In this specific case he was wrong. His wife, who eventually came for treatment with him, had not fallen out of love with her husband but did have some sexual inhibitions that needed to be addressed. However, his feeling that working to overcome a sexual difficulty is bound to bring out other unfinished business in a relationship is right on target. As a result, a man who senses that working on a sexual problem will bring to the fore bigger problems in the relationship may opt to keep the sexual problem rather than risk losing the relationship.

- *He knows he has a problem but is absolutely humiliated by the prospect of dealing with it directly or, worse yet, of going to a stranger and admitting his penis doesn't work.* Not surprisingly, this is perhaps the most common reason a man does not embrace resolving his problem with open arms. Most men are so embarrassed by their problems that it is easier for them simply to pretend they do not exist or to diminish their importance. Even more gut-wrenching is a powerful fear that a man may not be able to solve the problem even if he does work on it. With this emotional backdrop, it is little wonder that the average American male is likely to do everything he can to run way from the problem and will be willing to consider working on it only when he reaches the point of absolute desperation.

START TALKING

How then, do you determine if your partner is open to working on his sexual problem?

A lot of women make the mistake of second-guessing. Some assume their men will not do something when they will. Others wrongly interpret a discussion about the problem initiated by their partners as a surefire sign that they are willing to work on it.

The bottom line is that the only way to know if your partner will cooperate is to talk about it. And considering how sensitive he feels about having a sexual problem to begin with, the way you approach him can have a lot to do with the outcome.

The Right Time

As the saying goes, "timing is everything." If your timing is poor, there is only a slim chance that you are going to get the kind of response you are hoping to get.

The best way to promote a positive outcome is to set aside a special time in advance. I recommend that you let your partner know that there is something important, though not urgent, that you want to discuss and then negotiate a mutually agreeable time.

The worst times to bring up the problem are:

- During or after an argument
- When your partner is under a period of particularly high stress
- When either of you does not have the time to talk
- During or right after a lovemaking session.

This is an important point. Unless he wants to discuss the problem in bed, you shouldn't either, especially if the problem has existed for a while. In order to have a shot at getting your point across, your partner has to be in the right frame of mind to listen. Since a man is at his most vulnerable after a sexual failure, his impulse is to become defensive, which will make it likely that what you say will fall on deaf ears. If you have waited this long to bring it up, you can wait a little longer.

Of course, there are times when the lack of a response would be inappropriate. If you are in a new sexual relationship and things do not go well, or you are in a long-term relationship and a problem suddenly appears, or your partner is obviously upset, you are going to have to say something. Although it may still not be the right time to go into a full-length discussion, there are some things you can say that can help ease the moment.

- *Let him know you hear his frustration.* Conventional wisdom has it that when a man has a problem in bed, a woman should downplay the situation at the time that it occurs. But a lot of men have told me that when a partner simply says, "Don't worry about it," he perceives that he is not being heard and his feelings are being dismissed. "A lot of women think that telling a guy 'it doesn't matter' when he has a problem will make him feel better, but it doesn't," one man who often had a problem with his erection early in a relationship told me. "Telling a guy who feels as limp as his dick, 'Don't worry,' makes him feel like she doesn't understand how humiliating and frustrating the experience is."

What, then, should you say? Start by acknowledging his feelings. If it is clear that he is distressed, tell him that you can see how upset he is. A straightforward statement like "I know that you feel bad," or "I see how hard you're taking this," won't take the problem away, but it will validate how he feels. Resist the impulse to tell him you understand exactly how he feels, however, because unless you are male, you don't. You can tell him that you're sorry he feels as bad as he does, though.

- *If you are upset, don't lie.* He'll pick it up anyway. Letting your partner know that you feel a little frustrated or disappointed just makes you human and will not break his spirit. On the contrary, your honesty will reassure him that you are leveling with him and that you are not going to suddenly abandon him.

- *Let him know you will work on the problem with him.* This is really what he most needs to hear. After acknowledging how he feels and sharing your feelings with him, the best course of action is to direct your focus toward the future. If you are in a new relationship, a commitment on your part to take the necessary action to resolve the problem goes a long way toward alleviating a man's anxiety about being dumped because of the problem. If your relationship is long term and you have already made a commitment to working on the problem, restate your commitment. Reassure him that you love him and that the relationship is not threatened because of the problem.

In essence, if a response is called for, the tenor should be something like this: "I know that you are feeling really down that you came fast again, and in all honesty I wish you could last longer, too. But I care about you, so we'll work on it together." Then, when the two of you are out of the bedroom and more removed from the situation, you can set aside a more productive time to engage in an in-depth discussion.

Be Direct

If you want your partner to take your feelings about his problem seriously, you are going to need to bring it out into the open in a direct, no-nonsense way. This may seem obvious, but in fact, I have found that a lot of women who are with dysfunctional men keep stiff upper lips and make light of the problems. Some women are reluctant to bring the subject up because of their own shyness about discussing sexual issues. Other women are afraid to bring up the problems out of fear that it will put more pressure on their partners and only make the problems worse. Usually, though, what a woman fears is angering her partner or being met by an insensitive response to her concerns.

For whatever reason, if you do not confront the problem directly, if you meekly bring up the subject, immediately adding a "but"—"*but* it really doesn't matter," "*but* you don't need to worry about it," "*but* we don't have to talk about it if you don't want to"—or if you stew in silence, you are not doing yourself or your partner any favors. In fact, your relationship is likely to suffer. With the exception of a problem that appears early in a relationship as the result of anxiety, telling a man it doesn't matter is a flat-out lie. It does matter, and both of you know it. Pretending that there is no problem, or that it will disappear if you ignore it, or that you have no feelings about it will not make him feel better. It will not make you feel better either. On the contrary, the anger and frustration that you both are experiencing, if not openly addressed, will seep into your relationship in all sorts of insidious ways. If you do nothing, you are implicitly responsible for keeping the problem alive. By taking no action, you and your partner are colluding in an unspoken contract that says, "You don't have to look at this if you really don't want to." You can bet that given such an easy out, he is going to take it. Naturally, the result of such an agreement is the perpetuation of the problem.

What is the best way to encourage a constructive dialogue? Before anything, you need to let your partner know that you really care about him and that what you are about to share with him is not a negative statement about your relationship. The more confident a man feels that you love him despite the problem, the more likely he is to be open to listening to you.

I have found that after you give him some reassurance, the best way to get the least defensive responses is to state your feelings about the problem briefly in an assertive but nonaccusatory way. Here are a few examples:

- "Over the past few months I have noticed that you seem to have lost interest in sex. It concerns and upsets me. I feel rejected."
- "Because I am embarrassed about discussing this with you, I haven't brought it up before. When you come fast, it makes sex less pleasurable for me. Maybe it wouldn't be a problem for a woman who came more quickly, but it takes me more time. I know you would hold off if you could, and I would like to work toward doing that."
- "We've been dating for a while now, and I feel hurt and confused that you haven't approached me sexually. I wonder if you find me attractive or if something else is holding you back."

This introduction should immediately be followed with a questioning approach to engage him in the conversation. Here are some of the things you are going to want to ask:

- What are your feelings about the problem? How big a problem is this for you? Does it upset you?
- Have you always had the problem?
- Are you aware that there is help for the problem? Do you know that this is not an uncommon problem and that it can be solved?
- Have you ever thought about working on the problem? How would you feel about our working on the problem together?
- Is there anything that I am doing or not doing that's affecting you?

EXPECT RESISTANCE

Unless you are lucky, your partner is not going to be agreeable to working on the problem right off the bat. You may do a perfect job addressing the problem and still find yourself facing a man who sulks, or storms off, or is otherwise unreceptive to dealing with what you are telling him. This less than desirable response is never pleasant. But it's a lot easier to deal with if you expect it and don't overreact to it.

The first thing to do when encountering resistance is to let him vent his feelings without reacting negatively to them. Sometimes this can be difficult, particularly if he responds in anger or acts belligerently. It helps to keep in mind that his anger is almost always a defense, a way of covering up his pain and humiliation. If you are able to hear the anger as hurt, you will have an easier time listening to what is often a tirade. Also, if you do not react with anger yourself, he is likely to calm down more quickly.

The second step in overcoming resistance is to determine its source. Is he angry because you never brought it up before? Is he afraid he won't be able to solve the problem? Does he simply not care about you or the problem? Use the reasons why men don't want to solve their problem mentioned earlier as a kind of checklist, a way of confirming or ruling out possible reasons for the resistance. This will give you a good basis for evaluating whether or not working together is a reasonable possibility. As I discussed earlier, some forms of resistance are a direct offshoot of a man's unhappiness in his relationship. Unless these issues are resolved, working on the sexual problem will be fruitless. Obviously if he is not committed to the relationship or wants out of it, working on a sexual problem is out of the question. Bringing this fact to the surface will force you, as a couple, to deal with some unresolved issues between you that have been under cover until now.

If a problem in your relationship is not the source of the sexual problem, the third step in dealing with resistance is to work through it. This process is often fairly simple. For instance, if the main difficulty is his embarrassment about dealing openly with the sexual problem, some reassurance from you that you think no less of him because of the problem, coupled with your desire to solve it, is usually sufficient.

More often, though, you will have to spend a lot of time dealing with his resistance. Expect numerous discussions. Agree to table a conversation if it gets too overheated. You can always come back to it later. Find a way to keep things light. Smile, love, and be persistent.

During this initial period, which may take months, it is crucial not to vent your frustration in a negative way. If you are frustrated and feeling as if you are making no headway, you are likely to feel like lashing out in a last-ditch attempt to try to get your uncooperative partner to hear it your way. This is a mistake and only makes the problem worse.

Here are the kinds of things you are likely to feel like doing, but you should instead swallow your comments unsaid:

- *Never* compare him with other men you have been with. This can be very tempting, particularly if he insists that you are the only woman who has complained about his functioning. Unfortunately it is a tactic that invariably backfires and makes the problem worse.
- *Never* develop a running commentary on how he is doing during sex, even if what you have to say is occasionally positive. This will only increase his already intense anxiety about his performance.
- *Never* attack him or speak derogatorily about his sexual difficulty. According to the men I've worked with, women have a way of coming out with some real beauts that hit below the belt. Here are just a few choice examples: "So fast?" "Can't you control yourself?" "I've been with a lot of men, but none who have had this problem." "Is it in?"

As bitchy as these remarks sound, they are more the result of defensiveness and frustration than nastiness. A lot of women misinterpret their partners' problems as a reflection on themselves and their desirability and strike out in defense. And there is no more surefire way to score a hit than to demean a male's masculinity. Nevertheless, these remarks are very destructive to a man's already debilitated ego and are more likely to increase rather than reduce his resistance.

WHEN HE STILL REFUSES TO BUDGE

What if after you do all the above, he still says with actions or with words, "Forget it, I'm not going to deal with this."

Sometimes it is simply a matter of time. Many men I have worked with need to go through a process of accepting the problem and developing a willingness to deal with what often feels like an open wound. Others, particularly men with erection problems, need some time to convince themselves that the problems are not going to go away by themselves.

The more likely possibility, if you have an intact relationship, is that you are not taking a strong-enough position. You need to be very direct about the effect the problem is having on you and the consequences on the relationship if your partner does not work on the problem. Otherwise, he may not get the message, and you can end up in such a rage about his lack of responsiveness that your relationship will be destroyed.

A couple I recently worked with can attest to this. At our first meeting Cynthia, a woman in her early forties, told me that their sex life had finally come to a complete halt after two years of what she described as "begging" her husband, Craig, for sex. She was furious at him, she said, for having ignored her frequent complaints about what she viewed as his insufficient sexual desire. "I can't believe that it has taken two goddamn years to get him in here," she said.

"Why *did* it take so long for you to seek help?" I asked Craig, following his wife's lead.

Craig seemed genuinely perplexed. "To be truthful," he told me, "part of it was that I was embarrassed about talking about sex with a stranger. Also," he added quickly, "up until a month ago I honestly didn't realize how much it bothered Cynthia. It's true that she complained from time to time, but she complains about a lot of things. It was only when she said that she was thinking about ending the relationship that I realized that not having much sex was very upsetting to her."

"How can anyone be that dense?" Cynthia shot back snidely. "If your wife tells you that she doesn't feel she is getting enough sex, isn't it obvious how serious that is?"

The answer is no. Particularly when you are dealing with a sensitive issue that a man may prefer to avoid, it is not enough to "complain" from time to time. It is not enough to be a little bit upset. Although I would certainly not recommend opening your discussion with "If you do not work this out, our relationship is history," at some point you need to make it clear that you have no intention of living the rest of your life under the present conditions. And that point should come before you are so infuriated that you are ready to walk out the door.

I have worked with many women who, by the time they and their husbands get to me, are still in the relationship physically, but have long ago slammed the door behind them emotionally. That is exactly what happened in Cynthia's case. By the time she made Craig aware of her unhappiness and he was willing to work on the problem, Cynthia was so incensed that she decided to end the relationship.

What if, even after you take a strong position, your partner is still not willing to work on the problem? The next move is yours. Can you live with the problem? Can you live with his not dealing with the problem? What do you want to do vis-à-vis the relationship? These are questions that you need to ask and that only you can answer.

THE NEXT STEP: A ROAD MAP

Once you and your partner have made a commitment to solve the problem, you can begin working in a methodical way. The next three chapters are filled with exercises designed to deal with the problems I have discussed. The exercises in the following chapter should be done by everyone. The chapter after that focuses on techniques for dealing with premature ejaculation and erection problems. The final chapter is geared toward men with inhibitions and desire problems. Since some men have problems that overlap, I recommend that you read through all the chapters.

Even though the exercises are structured and can be very helpful if done properly, it is always important to keep in mind the discomfort your partner is feeling simply by virtue of having to work on his problem. If you become frustrated and disappointed, so will he. If you communicate that you are there for the duration, he will be more relaxed and his progress will move much more quickly.

8

Body Sex, Mind Sex, and Talking about Sex

If there is any one motto that summarizes the strategy for resolving most sexual problems, it is this: Think less and feel more. Whether a man has premature ejaculation, impotence, desire, or orgasm problems, there is so much noise in his head that he can't focus on what he is feeling in his body. This inability to concentrate on the present is a cornerstone of almost all sexual dysfunctions. Learning to get out of his head by tuning in to his body is the first step in successfully overcoming them.

This approach is called sensate focus. It is a very powerful tool. Staying in touch with the pleasurable physical sensations of the moment curbs the tendency of the mind to run ahead of the body, a problem found frequently among men with PE and erection problems. Being able to respond to good feelings in his body also gives a man who doesn't feel strong desire or sexual passion a way of functioning sexually. Finally, focusing on the present helps alleviate performance anxiety. If a man's attention is focused on *what* he is doing, he will worry less about *how* he is doing.

In this chapter you will learn how to help your partner make sex less related to what is going on in his mind and more connected to what he is feeling in his body. You will also learn to open up the lines of sexual communication. These skills are crucial to good sexual functioning and lay the foundation for dealing with the specific problems discussed in the next two chapters.

The exercises in this chapter should be done by everyone, regardless of the problem.

MIND SEX VS. BODY SEX

In a world of romance novels and porn flicks, it is easy to forget that in its most primitive form, sexual arousal is a physiological response to pleasurable physical stimulation. When four-year-old Johnny walks around with his hand on his crotch, he's not thinking that three-year-old Mary is a hot babe. He touches himself simply because it feels good. A male infant will get an erection if he is dried off after a bath by his mother or by a well-trained gorilla. He does not think: "Mommy is pretty and smells good, and the gorilla is hairy and disgusting." He just feels the sensation and responds to it.

The man who has a sexual problem has lost this primitive ability to become aroused by just feeling. Often that is because he has developed the habit of arousing from sexual fantasy or anticipation, imagining and thinking about sex instead of relating to what is actually happening. I call this hyperfantasizing.

Most men fantasize and do it often. The man who undresses you with his eyes is mentally arousing himself (and maybe you, too). The excitement that a man feels watching his partner become aroused is also a form of fantasy, a purely mental sexual experience. Then, of course, there are sexually explicit films and books that enrich a man's sex fantasy toolbox.

Am I saying that mental arousal is wrong, perverted, or a serious problem? Absolutely not. Mental stimulation, using words and pictures to heighten physical arousal, can make sex interesting and fun. Also, using fantasy may be necessary in helping a man with serious conflicts about sex overcome his anxiety. The problem is not fantasy per se, but that men with sexual problems use it to excess. The man with premature ejaculation tends to arouse mentally to such a degree that he becomes unable to exert control over the timing of his orgasm. He is oblivious of the relationship between his arousal and what is actually happening at any particular moment during sex. An excessive amount of mental stimulation is also a major factor in many cases of impotence. A man whose main source of arousal is mental is ripe for developing erection problems as he gets older and as sexy thoughts are no longer sufficient stimulation to produce or sustain an erection.

For a man with a desire or an orgasm problem, sex has become so much of a head trip that his need to fantasize is like an addiction. He is so out of touch with the physical aspect of arousal that if he becomes distracted, his fantasy does not click in at just the right moment, and his arousal disintegrates.

Mental arousal has another major glitch: While the mind can turn you on, it also can turn you off. One of the major distractions that makes it difficult for a man with a sexual problem to remain focused on what he is feeling in his body is anxiety. Once a man has developed a sexual problem, he spends a lot of time worrying about his performance. His mind is split: One part is focused on the task of the moment; the other sits in judgment about how well he is doing. The movie that runs through his head flip-flops between being tuned in to what he is feeling and worrying about his performance: Is his erection hard enough? Will he come fast enough? Will he come too fast? Is his partner enjoying herself? Too busy concentrating on *how* he is doing, he is unable to concentrate fully on *what* he is doing.

Learning to turn down the volume on the mental aspect of sex and raise the volume on the physical aspect is an important component of resolving many sexual problems. A man needs to tune in to what he is feeling in his body before he can have control over what his body is doing. When he is absorbed in pleasurable physical sensations, very little of his attention is left to judge his performance. If he concentrates on the physical feelings of penetration rather than thinking, "Wow, I'm doing it," he will not explode the second he goes inside.

For the man struggling with impotence, a sensate focus—arousing from pleasurable physical stimulation—gives him a consistent and reliable way of getting an erection. Rather than view his body as an uncooperative enemy, he begins to trust it to do what it is supposed to do.

Sensate focus also helps a man who is sexually inhibited or sexually unresponsive with a woman. With work and a strong desire to succeed, he can experience good sexual feelings with her if he can learn to appreciate the sensations that come from being touched in a sexual way.

OVERCOMING A MAN'S RESISTANCE
TO A PHYSICAL APPROACH TO SEX

Although helping a man develop a sensory approach to sex is the key to overcoming many sexual problems, convincing him to approach sex in a physical way may not be easy. Below are the most common forms of resistance that you will need to overcome, before you can begin practicing the exercises in this chapter.

- *Don't most normal men think about sex in this way?* For the heavy-duty fantasizer, viewing sex primarily as a physical activity seems completely alien. Explain that mental arousal is normal and positive but that he simply has been doing too much of a good thing. I will never forget Irv, a thirty-eight-year-old married man with children who had the mind of an adolescent. It was a miracle that Irv had not been killed by a car because he fantasized about everything in a skirt. He was in a perennial state of sexual anticipation, his mind running ahead to what he imagined would happen next. It was no surprise that Irv had one of the worst cases of premature ejaculation I ever treated.
- *How am I supposed to get aroused without using sexual thoughts?* A person who never learns to serve a tennis ball properly may, from time to time, get the ball over the net and in the right court by hitting the ball any old way. But without mastering the basics of a good service motion, he will never develop a reliable serve. In the same way, it is only by learning to arouse himself from the pleasurable physical sensations in his

body that a man will develop a consistent basis for good sexual functioning.

- *If I stay in the moment and focus on the sensations, won't I come too fast?* This question, which is asked almost exclusively by premature ejaculators, comes from the understandable but faulty belief that the best way to last longer is to focus on everything else *but* what is happening in his body. It can take a man a little while to understand that he first needs to be in touch with what he is feeling in his body before he can control it.

  A lot of my patients have found this idea easier to grasp when I compare developing ejaculatory control with how a child develops bladder control. Just as the first step in learning to not pee in your pants is learning to identify the sensations associated with urinating, the first step in developing good ejaculatory control is being able to feel the sensations that let you know you are getting close to orgasm.

- *Sex doesn't feel as good as it used to.* Even after the problem is solved, many premature ejaculators have this complaint. Instead of coming whenever he feels like it, the man now has to work at control, to concentrate on it. From his point of view, things are not as much fun as before. Also, if he views orgasm as the best part of sex, he may not be into delayed gratification.

  For a mature man, this frame of mind is usually temporary. In time his ability to have control will become more automatic. Eventually he will also reach the point where lasting longer will in and of itself become more pleasurable to him. As a result, his motivation to control his ejaculation will increase.

  In many ways the process is similar to getting into the habit of working out. When first beginning an exercise program, a lot of people virtually have to drag themselves to the gym. Eventually, as they begin to reap the benefits, they are motivated to exercise because it makes them feel good.

- *I do not like being touched.* Men who feel this way often have body image issues. A man who does not like certain parts of his body—his love handles, his flabby arms, his sunken chest, his small penis—will often feel self-conscious about having these parts touched. The best way to overcome this is to talk about the parts of your body that you are less than enamored with. It also helps to let your partner know that you think he's fine the way he is—even if he isn't perfect.

Another more insidious reason why a man may react adversely to being touched is that he has been physically abused. And unless you spot this resistance and work with your partner to overcome it, you will make very little progress in resolving his problem.

Fear of being touched that is the result of physical abuse is easily recognized. Here are a few things to look for: A man who has been physically abused will become very tense when the part of his body that has been hit is touched. He will also be very anxious at the prospect of being touched in a sensual way and will do everything that he can to steer the exercises away from his being touched and toward his touching you. If he has the ability to tolerate being touched and has not pushed you away, chances are that you will notice him grimacing or experience him as very distant when you are touching him.

You can begin helping your partner overcome his resistance to being touched and responding to sex in a physical way by telling him that he is always in charge. He always has permission, at any time, to stop you when he feels threatened or uncomfortable. Progress can be made, but it will be slow.

All these signals are cause for concern and you should ask your partner about abuse in his background before continuing. If he shares with you, or you have any reason to suspect, that he has been sexually abused, *do not continue with the exercises!* A person with a history of sexual abuse can experience a psychotic episode if he is confronted with any of the triggers of the original abuse. Although men who have been sexually abused can be helped, it should always be under the supervision of a therapist.

Once you explain the difference between mental and physical arousal to your partner and have dealt with his preliminary resistance, you are ready to begin. The following guidelines apply to all the exercises in this book:

1. Each exercise should be done at least once. You should move forward only when you have mastered the prior exercise.
2. Read the exercise two or three times. Imagine it mentally as you read. You're going to be in charge, so it is important that you know what you're doing. Also, discuss the exercise with your partner before doing it. Make sure he knows what is going to occur and understands its purpose.
3. Set aside a special time each week to practice. Most people's lives are so hectic that if you leave the timing to chance, you will never find time.
4. You and your partner should not expect that he is going to do everything correctly the first time. The freer he feels to make errors and learn from them, the faster his progress will be. The more concerned he is with getting everything right, the less focused he will be on the task at hand.
5. Try to keep things light. Smile. Have a good time. Taking things too seriously is a mistake. Whatever happens in any particular encounter is not important. It is the overall trend that counts.
6. Resolving any sexual problem requires that a man recognize when he is not focused on the moment. When this happens, he should simply relax and refocus. Anytime he feels nervous, anxious, or distracted, a little red flag should go up, alerting him that he's not on the right track. When this happens, he should stop, breathe deeply, and think: "Stop thinking about whether you're doing this right, how sexy she is, how foolish you look, or if you're getting an erection. Focus on the physical sensations that you're experiencing in your body right now."

It is very important that he talk to himself in precisely this way. That's because if he thinks, "Stop being nervous," he will become fixated on how nervous he is and become more uptight. Try it yourself.

If I tell you, "Stop thinking about pink elephants," what comes to mind? Pink elephants, of course. But if you tell yourself, "Stop thinking about those pink elephants and focus on red giraffes," your attention will shift to the latter.

Your partner may need to use this self-talk frequently at first, particularly as the exercises become more sensual. That's okay. The more aware he is of when he is out of the moment, the faster he will learn how to refocus his attention.

LEARNING TO RELAX: THE FIRST STEP

Have you ever noticed that when you become tense, you lose control over what is going on in your body? The inability to relax can cause you to miss a tennis shot because you are thinking about how important it is to win the next point rather than focusing on the ball. Anxiety can make you oblivious of your surroundings. In cases of extreme fright or panic, you lose control over voluntary bodily functions.

In the same way a man whose anxiety is through the roof will not be able to concentrate on physical sensations. Developing the ability to relax in anxiety-producing situations is so critical that unless your partner is able to relax by mastering the following exercises, it will be very difficult for him to make any real progress. Without relaxation, there can be no focus.

Below are a series of relaxation exercises. Although your partner may prefer one form of breathing to another, he should be familiar with all the techniques. It is especially important that he master deep breathing and develop some relaxing imagery since he will be using these techniques throughout the exercises in this part of the book.

EXERCISE 1: Deep Breathing, Yoga Style

Facing your partner, sit comfortably on the floor with your legs crossed. It is best if you both sit straight without leaning on anything. However, if either of you has a back problem, position yourself so that you are leaning against a wall, bed, or couch.

Ask your partner to close his eyes. Then tell him to breathe through his nose, very slowly, while you count. He should feel the air going in and filling up his abdomen. This is very important. Many people tend to breathe shallowly into the chest, making them feel more tense and possibly leading to hyperventilation.

Count to six when inhaling, to four when exhaling. As you exhale, you feel the tension being drained from your body. Be sure to pause a second between breaths. Make sure that when he breathes, his abdomen is rising and falling with each breath. Do the breathing with him. It is important for you to relax, too.

Now have him place his left hand on his abdomen and his right hand on his chest. Gently put your hand over his right hand and tell him to breathe deeply in a way that pushes your hand up. The inhalation and exhalation should be slow, even, and relaxed. Some people find it useful to imagine a wave going through the chest and into the abdomen and then slowly being pulled away like the tide. Have him repeat the exercise with your hand over his for as long as it takes for him to begin feeling comfortable with the breathing.

His breathing should not be forced. If he is taking each breath as if it were his last, he is working too hard. Chances are he is also holding his breath after inhaling. Explain that the breathing should be rhythmical and unforced.

If his chest is rising as much as, or more than, his abdomen, as you and he can notice by observing his right hand, he is breathing too shallowly. To get him more familiar with the feeling of breathing abdominally, remove your hand and place a book on his abdomen. Have him repeat the exercise trying to raise the book. Eventually he will come to experience the difference between breathing through his chest and breathing through his diaphragm.

Besides doing this with you, he should practice the breathing for five to ten minutes each day on his own. With practice, he should begin to feel the calming effect of deep breathing.

EXERCISE 2: Synchronized Breathing

This is a wonderful way for a couple to relax together as well as to learn how to be physically close and intimate without being sexual.

Begin by lying down with both of you facing the same direction and the person in front curling his or her body into the body of the person behind. The person to the rear then puts his or her hands on the other's abdomen. The idea is for the two of you to inhale and exhale at the same time. Breathe together for about five minutes. Then switch places and repeat the exercise. You should feel relaxed, even sleepy when you are finished.

If your partner becomes aroused, he isn't focused on the breathing, pure and simple. Repeat the exercise, suggesting that he think more about the air going in and out of his lungs than his penis going in and out of your vagina. Then try the exercise again. If you and your partner enjoy it, try this form of relaxation before starting each of the exercises. The important thing is to relax and have fun.

EXERCISE 3: Deep Breathing Combined with Relaxed Imagery

The first step is to develop a relaxing image. Have your partner think about a time and place when he was totally relaxed or a time and place that would be most relaxing. Ask him to describe the scene. Use color, making it as real as possible in his mind. He can have more than one if he wants. They're free.

Next, go back to breathing deeply, and have your partner think of the relaxing images he has developed. Be persistent. The full relaxing effort of these techniques takes time to develop. Practice.

The next step is to combine a man's newfound ability to relax with mental images of sexual activity he finds anxiety-producing. Work with him on developing a sexual scenario—real or imagined—and identifying each particular part of the situation where he finds his anxiety increasing as he thinks about it.

Begin with a few minutes of relaxed deep breathing. The idea is for him to be able to "see" the sexual episode in his head, to stop the image when he gets to a part he is uncomfortable with, and to switch mentally to the relaxing imagery. After a few minutes he should continue with the sexual scene he's imagining, stopping again and returning to the relaxing imagery if his anxiety returns.

It is important that your partner master this exercise because it will be very helpful in reducing his nervousness during the exercises discussed later on.

LEARNING TO FOCUS HIS ATTENTION

Now that your partner has started to learn how to relax in the face of anxiety, he can begin learning to concentrate his attention on the action that is happening when you have sex. Being able to focus on the momentary sensory experience will help prevent his mind from hopping ahead. Concentrating on what he is doing will also reduce his worry about how well he is doing. After all, if you are concentrating on what you are doing, you aren't obsessing about how you're doing.

The following exercises are useful for all dysfunctions. The goal of each is to help a man learn to concentrate his attention on the sensations he is feeling in his body during sex. Since most men with sexual problems are completely out of touch with what it means to be absorbed in touch, sight, and smell, I have found that it is a good idea first to familiarize them with the experience in a nonsexual way. Then they can move on to activities that are more sensual.

EXERCISE 1: Staying in the Here and Now:
A Nonsexual Beginning

Gather together three objects that have different forms, shapes, and textures. Have your partner sit down and shut his eyes. Now place one of the objects in his hand. Ask him to feel it, taking his time, and describe what he feels. Is it rough? Is it smooth? Is it light or heavy? Is it cool, hot? What is its shape? Does the shape change?

Once he is able to get the hang of it, ask him to explore your hand and arm in the same way, describing what it feels like to touch. Make sure he takes his time and really explores.

If he rushes through the exercise or keeps opening his eyes, he is probably wondering if he is doing it correctly. If this happens, have him relax and refocus on just the physical sensations and nothing else.

Next, with his eyes closed, touch his arm with the various objects in front of you. Ask him to describe what he is feeling. Is it a ticklish touch? Is it rough? Does it feel sharp? Heavy?

After using several objects, you can begin touching his arm with your hands. Massage one of his fingers, and ask him to describe what it feels like. Use a pitter-patter motion up and down his arm, and see if he can describe that. Finally, stroke his arm in a feathery way, and ask him to describe what that feels like. You know he is on track if he can accurately discriminate between different sensations.

If, on the other hand, he can't interpret or describe what he is feeling or says, "It doesn't feel like anything," he's missing the point. This response is common among men who use fantasy a lot. That's because they tend to dichotomize sensations. "Good" sensations are feelings associated with arousal and orgasm. Sensations not directly related to sexual arousal are perceived as "nothing." For a man like this to make progress, he needs to understand that a touch can be pleasurable without being sexual.

EXERCISE 2: Nonsexual Massage

Once he gets the hang of how to keep his attention where the action is, you can move on to more sensual touching.

Begin by lying nude either on the bed or on the floor. You should be on your stomach with your eyes closed. Slowly, and in a relaxed way, ask your partner to start massaging your extremities—your toes, feet, hands, head. Then ask him to begin working on the center of your body. Have him massage your shoulders, then move down your back to your legs and calves.

Turn over, and ask him to repeat the process of massaging the front of your body. He may touch your breasts in a nonsexual way but should completely avoid your genitals. When he is done, lie quietly for a few minutes.

Repeat the whole process with him receiving.

If his touch seems tentative when he is giving, he is probably worrying about how well he is touching you and if you are enjoying it. If this happens, remind him that he is supposed to be focused on what he is feeling as he touches you rather than on what you are feeling.

Also, give him direct feedback as he massages you. Providing him with guidance in a noncritical way will help build his confidence in his ability to please you.

He's off the track if his touch seems sexual or you notice an erection or pre-ejaculation when you are finished. If this happens, have him repeat the exercise, verbalizing what he is feeling both as he is touching you and when you are touching him. Most men have an easier time staying focused while receiving a massage than giving one. Doing some deep breathing if he does feel himself become excited will also help him refocus, as will using the self-talk technique described earlier. Closing his eyes and imagining a relaxing situation in order to eliminate the visual arousal can help, too. Try different combinations until he finds one that works for him. The important thing is that he find a way to relax and experience nonsexual physical sensations.

What if you notice that his body seems tense and he is unable to relax? If he has PE, he may be concerned that he will get an erection. Remind him that, rather than try not to become aroused, it is preferable to become aroused, recognize that he is jumping ahead, and then refocus his attention. Repeat the exercise until he can simply enjoy receiving your touch without worrying and without getting turned on.

If your partner flinches when you touch him, this is a good indication that he was abused at one time. If you suspect the abuse was sexual, do not continue. You can, however, proceed with caution if you know the abuse was physical and not sexual. It is crucial that your partner always feel he is in control and that he has permission to stop when he feels too uncomfortable. At that point you should have him do the deep breathing exercise combined with relaxed imagery. Once he has relaxed, you can begin touching him again, although don't be surprised if at first you need to stop often.

EXERCISE 3: Playing Blind Children

Years ago I had the unique experience of meeting a blind little boy. Unable to see me, he proceeded to feel my face, nostrils, ears, and mouth with the kind of unabashed inquisitiveness that I had never before experienced. As he described to me what he was feeling, I was amazed to learn that he, in three minutes, knew more about the contours of my face than I knew about them my whole life. In the following exercise you and your partner will learn about each other's bodies in a similar way.

Start by sitting opposite each other with your legs crossed. Since your partner may have a tendency to mimic you, it is a good idea for him to go first. With his eyes closed, have him begin by touching your hair and working his way down your body, describing what he is feeling as if he were taking in all the information about your shape through his hands. Have him try to imagine that he is "seeing you" through his fingertips for the first time. Ask him to describe each part in terms of its texture, temperature, and shape. It is okay for him to touch your genitals briefly, but he should not focus on them.

As he touches, ask him to verbalize what he is feeling. A man who uses mental arousal excessively tends to have a lot of trouble staying with what he is actually feeling physically. Describing what you feel like, step by step, will help him stay in the moment and refocus when he jumps ahead. If he starts describing your upper arm in sensual or sexual terms, he's got it wrong. Ask him to focus on texture, form, and size. Ask him to tell you what he can taste or smell without any sexual commentary.

You should be concerned if he seems to be somewhere else while touching you. This is a sure sign that he is suppressing his arousal. A man who is very self-conscious about doing things right and is afraid that this exercise will excite him is likely to try to control his arousal. He does this by trying to distract himself by thinking about the un-sexiest of thoughts: sports, what he has to do at work tomorrow, dirty laundry—virtually anything that will keep his mind off the fact that he is touching an attractive female or is being touched by her.

If you do not catch his tendency to overcontrol his arousal early and correct it, the result can be disastrous. Once again you need to explain to him that it is a lot better if he gets aroused and then uses self-talk and breathing to refocus than to take himself out of the moment and experience no arousal at all.

Then do the same to him. Make sure that you go over his whole body, head to toe, paying as much attention to his feet as to his chest.

Make sure to take your time, slowly exploring each part of his body as if he were a piece of sculpture. Verbalize what you feel, just as he did.

You can move on when he is able to enjoy doing the exercise without becoming aroused. It also helps if you've learned to enjoy focusing on the sensation of touch, too.

EXERCISE 4: Finding the Tape

Take three pieces of nonstick tape, and hide them on inconspicuous parts of his body. Turn out the lights, have him close his eyes, and tell your partner that his job is to discover where the tape is. The game does not end until he has found all three pieces. This will force him to concentrate on the here and now.

EXERCISE 5: Name That Thing

This exercise helps a man focus on genital sensations and reinforces the idea that he can have his penis touched without becoming overly anxious or overly aroused. It is also a terrific ego boost because most men are able to do it well even though they are initially convinced that there is no way they will be able to do it successfully. "How can I possibly not get aroused when my penis is being touched?" is a common response. I usually remind a patient that he touches his penis when he goes to urinate without getting an instant hard-on every time.

Have your partner lie on the floor or on the bed faceup and with his eyes closed. Tell him that you are going to touch his penis with different objects—nothing sharp. Ask him to describe how the different objects feel and then to guess what each object is. In order to make the exercise fun and interesting, be creative in your selection of items. A combination of Handi Wipes, a spoon, a piece of fruit with fleshy skin, such as an orange, and a small makeup or paint brush makes for interesting variation.

Most men have a lot of fun with this exercise, and to their amazement they do not get turned on. The exception is a man with extreme premature ejaculation. Actually he is not really aroused but is experiencing a knee-jerk response to having his genitals touched.

When this happens, have him breathe and refocus until his erection begins to dissipate. Then you can begin again.

If he has an erection problem and is totally unable to focus on what he is feeling, he probably has a heavy dose of performance anxiety. If he perceives his penis as small when it's flaccid, he may feel very self-conscious. Either way, have him practice his favorite relaxation technique until he can refocus.

EXERCISE 6: Advanced Sensuality: Body Touring

In this exercise you and your partner will learn to stay focused sensually even though contact is more sexual. Both of you will also have the opportunity to begin sharing how you enjoy being touched.

Keep in mind that with the exception of his genitalia, your partner probably does not have the foggiest idea of how he likes being touched. Men in general are fairly out of touch with their own sensuality. This is particularly true for men with sexual problems. Therefore, he should feel free to explore and experiment. Often women are not in tune with their own sensuality, either. If this is true for you, this exercise will be a terrific learning experience for you as well.

You should go first. Have your partner sit with his legs apart, leaning restfully against the back of the bed or couch. Position yourself so that you are sitting in between his legs with your back resting on his chest and your head positioned comfortably. Then take one of his hands, put your hand over his, and guide him slowly over your body, letting him know by the way you move his hand, the pressure you put on his hand, and where you move his hand how you enjoy being touched.

Some men have difficulty relinquishing control, so it is important that you tell him that from the outset you will be guiding him. His hand should be limp so you can move it easily. Cover your whole body, including breasts and genitals, but don't focus on these parts more than on any other.

After you have gone over your whole body, switch positions, and have him guide your hand over his body. Once you both are done, share your feelings about the exercise as well as what you have learned.

If he confesses that he was bored or learned nothing, this signals that he is not being very communicative about his preferences. In some instances he may be so out of touch with his sensuality that he just isn't able to differentiate one touch from another. If this is the case, continue the exercise until he begins to learn what feels good to him.

More likely, he does have some preferences but is embarrassed about communicating them to you. If he is inhibited about telling you what feels good sensually, you can bet he will have even more difficulty when it comes to communicating what he enjoys sexually.

LEARNING TO TALK ABOUT SEX

It is virtually impossible to have a good sex life, let alone resolve a sexual problem, without adequate communication about sexual likes and dislikes. Yet many people—men and women—are often hesitant to communicate openly about sexual matters. This tendency is intensified in the man for whom sex has become a sore spot.

Why would a man resist telling you about his sensual and sexual preferences? There are a number of reasons.

- *He thinks that if he were "normal," whatever his partner does to him would be sufficient.* Many men believe that they should not need to be stimulated in a specific way in order to function. This is particularly true if they think that the women they are with are experienced sexually. As one man suffering from an erection problem put it, "If her touch works for other guys and she's been with a lot of other guys, then I feel there must be something wrong with me if it doesn't work for me."
- *He feels that some of his requests will be seen as wimpy or unmasculine.* Many men have told me that they enjoy having their nipples sucked or licked or that they really like a lot of foreplay. Very few of these men ever communicate their preferences to their partners because they feel "that stuff is a girl thing," as one patient put it.

- *A man is often afraid of offending his partner if he asks her to do something she is not doing or to do something differently.* It is not uncommon for a man to tell me that he has not shared some important information about what he enjoys sexually out of fear of hurting his partner's ego. This is particularly true if a man suspects his partner feels somewhat responsible for the problem. "My girlfriend already feels undesirable because I have trouble with my erections, even though I have tried to explain to her that I've had this problem all my adult life," a forty-seven-year-old man told me. "So how do I tell her that her touch is too heavy-handed for me or that she doesn't stimulate my penis in as pleasing a way as she could? I'm afraid if I say anything, it will make her feel even more rejected."
- *A woman is supposed to be a mind reader.* A lot of men and women are guilty of somehow expecting their partners automatically to know what they want. This comes from a childlike perception that if someone really loves and cares about you, he or she will automatically know what you want, just as a mother is supposed intuitively to know her infant's needs. This mind-set can create many problems. When a man expects his partner to know what to do and when to do it and she does not respond in the way he expects, he may become angry. He may even begin to blame her for his sexual problem.

Just how inhibited can a man be? Barry is a good example. In his early forties, Barry is a successful businessman who suffers from a desire disorder. He had been married to Ellen for twenty years, yet there were many basic sexual facts of life that had never been discussed. When I asked Barry if Ellen had orgasms, he was uncertain, although he believed she probably did not, at least not with him. When I asked Barry if Ellen had orgasms when she masturbated, this otherwise sophisticated man looked at me as if I had just asked him if his wife enjoyed being strung up from the ceiling by her ankles. Barry had never seen or even asked Ellen whether she masturbated, let alone whether or not she had orgasms when she did. This was a clear indication that Barry and Ellen were not communicating on a sexual level. Barry had never even communicated to Ellen some very simple sexual preferences. It was only after months of therapy that Barry was able to tell his wife that having his testicles gently cupped was a tremendous turn-on for him. And it was only after considerable urging on my part that he finally confronted Ellen about the orgasm issue. Their mutual level of embarrassment was obvious from Barry's recounting of their discussion.

"My therapist told me to ask you if you masturbate to orgasm, and if so, how often do you do it?" he queried Ellen one night.

Ellen was too embarrassed to respond, and Barry, given his shyness, allowed the moment to slip away. A full week later, seemingly out of the blue, Ellen replied, "I'm not saying that I do, but if I did, it would happen about twice a week." Once this issue was out in the open, this totally changed their basic assumptions about sexual communication. Now that it had been established that she had orgasms, they were able to begin working on helping Ellen become more responsive to Barry. As she became more sexually responsive, his desire for her increased.

Whatever the reasons, a lack of communication about sexual issues can create havoc in relationships. Working through a sexual problem requires explicitness about sexual wants and needs. Even if there is no sexual problem, an inability to share with your partner how and where you like being touched makes sex less pleasurable.

Of course, communication about preferences is a two-way street. Up to this point I have been focused on helping a man inform his partner about his likes. But letting him know how and where you enjoy being caressed is also important. A lot of men are very inexperienced when it comes to touching a woman in a pleasing way. Their lack of finesse can create a number of problems. First, if a man is insecure about his ability to arouse his partner, he is likely to exert a lot of energy thinking about how he is doing when he should be focused on what he is feeling. Then again, he may think that he is perfectly adept when the truth is, he is a sexual klutz. If you feel that he is pawing at you in a displeasing manner, it will be almost impossible for you to sustain any real motivation to work with him. Fortunately this problem is easily remedied. Unlike sexual problems over which there is usually no conscious control, touching is a voluntary action.

Below are a series of exercises that can help.

EXERCISE 1: Female Anatomy Lesson

An adult version of "I'll show you mine if you show me yours," this exercise is intended to familiarize your partner with the different parts of your genitals and how each part functions. You will also be showing your partner how a man's genitals and a female's genitals, despite the obvious differences in appearance, are more alike than they are different.

Let the fainthearted beware! If you find yourself too embarrassed to do this exercise, chances are that you are a contributing factor in your partner's sexual problem. It is difficult for a man to feel comfortable with a woman's body if she is not comfortable with it herself.

Before doing this exercise, you should be freshly bathed. A natural douche is also a good idea to help you feel clean.

The anatomy lesson can be done in any room of the house where there is sufficient light. Explain that you want your partner to explore your genitals in a great deal of detail—by looking, touching, smelling, tasting—but that the exploration should be done in a nonsexual way. He should imagine that he is a medical student learning about this part of the body as he might any other.

You should be in a sitting-up position. Most women find it more comfortable to have something behind them for support, such as a wall or headboard or couch. Spread your legs wide, and have your partner lie down with his head between them. Begin by showing him the outer lips (labia majora) and inner lips (labia minora). Explain that the inner lips are the female analogue of the skin on a man's scrotum. Like the skin on the scrotum, the lips are very pliable.

Then gently pull away the skin that covers your clitoris. Like the penis, the clitoris has a foreskin. Show him exactly where the clitoris is, and have him touch it. Let him know that too direct a stroke can be irritating because the head of the clitoris is filled with highly sensitive nerve endings like the head (glans) of the penis.

Next, ask him to put his finger slowly into your vagina. Explain that if he presses his finger forward and upward, the spongy area he is feeling is the Grafenberg, or G, spot. Since the sensitivity of this area varies greatly from woman to woman, it will be helpful for you to let him know whether pressure in that spot is arousing or not. And unless your G spot is extremely sensitive, this is a good time to let him know that simply moving his finger in and out of the vagina with no clitoral stimulation will not help you climax.

Finally, have him taste the secretion from your vagina after removing his finger and smelling your genitals. (If you have never done this yourself, make sure you do so before doing this exercise.) Ask him to tell you his feelings about the smell and taste. Most men enjoy both, and chances are he will tell you that you taste and smell just fine. But if he has a negative reaction, he may be suffering some degree of genital aversion. If this is the case, the desensitization exercises in Chapter 10 will help you.

You might also want to use the opportunity to let your partner know how you enjoy having your genitals stimulated during this exercise. Since showing him is the best teacher, you can masturbate to orgasm while he watches if you feel comfortable doing it. Otherwise, talk through the way that you touch yourself. Praise him for things he is already doing right, and give him pointers for things that he is either not doing or not doing well.

EXERCISE 1(a): Male Anatomy Lesson

Now it's his turn. Take a good look at your partner's genitals. Have your partner familiarize you with the glans or head, the ridge, and the shaft. Touch each part, and feel the differences. Look at and feel the scrotum. Discover which testicle is larger. Notice if one testicle is lower than the other. Feel the skin on the scrotal sac, and note how similar it feels to your own inner vaginal lips.

After your partner goes through his show-and-tell, he can stimulate himself to orgasm while you watch if he wants to. If he's uncomfortable masturbating while you watch, have him describe to you how he enjoys having his genitals touched. Don't forget to ask if and how he enjoys having his testicles fondled.

EXERCISE 2: Shipwrecked

Pretend that you have been shipwrecked and swept ashore on a deserted island. Your partner, the sole island inhabitant, has not seen a woman in ten years. You should be totally passive. It is your partner's job to arouse you. You can let him know that he is capturing your interest only by movement and sound. If he is completely missing the boat, you can silently guide his hand to just the right place. The goal is not for you to have an orgasm but simply to be stimulated in a sexual way.

Repeat the same exercise with him being shipwrecked. After you are done, talk about your experience, sharing what you both liked, disliked, and would like more of.

EXERCISE 3: Shipwrecked to Orgasm

This exercise will give a man the necessary guidance so he can regularly bring you to orgasm with his hand or his mouth. Having a sexual problem is devastating to a man's ego. It is that much more horrendous if he feels that using his penis is the only way he can please you. On the other hand, if he has confidence that he can satisfy you in other ways, his anxiety about how well his equipment is working will be reduced.

Begin with you being passive. Let your partner know that this time his mission is not only to arouse you but to help you come. Using verbal as well as nonverbal clues, including putting your hand over his if necessary, gently guide him until he can successfully help you to an orgasm. Over time he should be able to bring you to an orgasm repeatedly with increasingly less direction from you.

If he doesn't seem to be getting the message after many attempts, there is a good chance that you are not communicating what you like very clearly to him. If this is the case, showing him is the best remedy. When you're ready, take his finger, place in on your clitoris, place your hand on top of his hand, and show him how fast and how hard or soft you like it touched.

If he still doesn't get it, either he is too anxious about performance to pay attention to what you're telling him or he has an aversion to a woman's genitals and just doesn't like to put his hand there. If it is the former, you need to let him know that you are not going to run out on him if he does not get it right away. If it is the latter, he needs to do the exercises in Chapter 10 so that he can neutralize his revulsion.

Finally, he might just be a sexual klutz. There is little that you can do about this other than to keep working with him again and again until he gets it right. Eventually he will, although he will probably never win an award for stud of the year.

EXERCISE 4: The Wish List

This exercise provides a structured way of giving you and your partner permission to ask for what each of you wants. On a piece of paper that you fold up and place in a hat, you and your partner write down five sensual wishes and five sexual wishes. Then, over the course of a number of weeks, the two of you agree to pick one wish when you are together until all the wishes have been fulfilled. A wish can include anything from a foot massage to oral sex to acting out a fantasy. However, both of you need to feel free not to fulfill a particular wish if it is very uncomfortable for you. If this is the case, talk about what it is about the wish that is making you or your partner uneasy. If either of you thinks that the wish is reasonable and your partner's response is unreasonable, compromise, be understanding, or start talking about getting help.

EXERCISE 5: A Contract to Communicate

Agree that as long as it takes for the two of you to become comfortable talking about sex, you will each communicate something that is pleasing to you and something that you would like to have your partner do or change after every sexual encounter. Continue doing this in a structured way until the ability to communicate about sex becomes second nature. Don't talk about problems during or right after sex. Wait until an agreed-on time. Be clear and direct, and don't forget to smile.

PREPARING TO MOVE FORWARD

The exercises in this chapter will give you a terrific foundation for a positive sex life. But just because you are progressing doesn't mean that you should consider these exercises a thing of the past. On the contrary, what you have learned provides the building blocks for all that is to come. If you get stuck as you move on, it may help for you to repeat the exercises you have just learned about in this chapter.

9

Overcoming Premature Ejaculation and Erection Problems

This chapter is geared toward dealing with premature ejaculation and erection problems caused by ignorance, performance anxiety, temporary physical problems, and changes in sexual functioning as a result of aging. Impotence that results from deeply rooted difficulties will not be responsive to sex therapy until the underlying conflict causing the problem has been resolved.

Although the goal of each exercise is different, depending on which problem a man has, the exercises are similar or identical. This may surprise you at first, but if you think about it, it makes a lot of sense.

A man with either premature ejaculation or impotence is out of tune with his body. For him to overcome either of these problems, he needs to get in touch with what is happening physically to him during sex so that he can begin to respond in a normal fashion. A man with premature ejaculation often develops an orgasm reflex that always occurs at, or shortly after, the point of penetration, regardless of how aroused he actually is physically. A man who is struggling with his erections frequently experiences an almost reflexive anxiety when he thinks he should be getting an erection or when penetration seems imminent.

Getting him in touch with the physical sensations of sex involves helping him become more sensitive to some things and less to others. A man with premature ejaculation, for example, needs to become desensitized to the anticipatory anxiety he feels about sexual contact, while becoming increasingly sensitized to what he is experiencing in his body. Someone who does not get a reliable erection needs to become desensitized to fluctuations in his level of arousal. At the same time, he needs to become more sensitive to the physical sensations that produce pleasure.

To help reduce anxiety, the exercises have been structured so that each step forward is small. Resist the impulse to skip any of the exercises. If you move too fast, you are likely to be met by failure and frustration. Patience, persistence, and a positive attitude will pay off.

Since these problems sometimes occur together, it is important to understand that if a man has both premature ejaculation and erection problems, *he must resolve the erection problem first.* There is no way that he will be able to focus on developing control when he is worried about getting it up. When this is the case, begin with the exercises for erection problems on page 236. When he has made sufficient progress with his erections, you can return to the exercises designed for ejaculatory control that follow.

There are two types of sensitization and desensitization exercises in this chapter.

Penile touch desensitization and sensitization: Here your partner will learn to reduce his anxiety and reflexive response to having his genitals touched while becoming more sensitive to the physical sensations he is experiencing.

Penetration desensitization and sensitization: The goal of these exercises is to get your partner to resolve the difficulties he has been experiencing around the anticipation of and actual experience of penetration. He will learn to experience intercourse as more pleasurable and less laden with anxiety. A man who comes too fast will learn how to develop control by focusing on the sensations of the moment. A man with erection problems will learn that the best way to sustain an erection is to rely on what he is feeling in his body.

BEWARE OF SELF-MONITORING

Of course, accomplishing all this is more easily said than done. Even though the exercises in the prior chapter provides an excellent foundation for helping a man relax and focus, the more sexually advanced exercises in this chapter are likely to trigger a great deal of anxiety about how he is doing.

This "spectatoring" or self-monitoring makes it much more difficult for him to focus on the sexual pleasure of the moment. Mentally he is stepping outside the sexual activity, observing and judging his performance, rather than focusing on what he is doing. Self-monitoring also feeds on itself. Once a man begins to monitor himself, he tends to become more and more tense, and this naturally limits his ability to function.

Knowing when a man is monitoring himself and what to do about it is crucial. Look for signs of tension. You may notice that he is tensing his abdominal muscles or clenching his fists or keeping his legs or feet rigid. His breathing may become shallow. He may even begin holding his breath.

You also may have a sense that he has become detached, that he is no longer "there" with you. If he has an erection problem, he may be praying for an erection to return or maybe he has begun wildly fantasizing in an effort to get his penis to respond. He may even begin looking at his penis periodically or touching it to ascertain its state of rigidity. If he has PE, he's probably thinking something like "baseball, baseball, baseball" because he's worried about coming too fast. Whatever he is doing, he is certainly not experiencing the sexual pleasure of the moment.

Another sign that he is monitoring himself is that he is shifting all the focus to you. A man like this often goes into the partner-pleasuring mode in an attempt to take the attention off his own performance.

When any signs of self-monitoring are present, you need to stop what you are doing and help your partner relax. It also helps if you don't take things too seriously. Everything will be all right. If you lighten up about the problem, he will too.

EXERCISES FOR PREMATURE EJACULATION

Overcoming premature ejaculation requires that a man become increasingly attuned to the sensations he experiences as he becomes aroused. This helps sensitize him to his level of arousal and makes it possible for him to adjust the pace of the sexual activity so that he can better control the timing of his orgasm. The first step in this process is to develop control with sensual and sexual activities that do not include intercourse. Once he is confident that he can voluntarily choose when to come with manual or oral stimulation, he can move on to the exercises that include intercourse.

The partner exercises should be done three times a week if possible, and the masturbation assignment twice a week. You should avoid intercourse during the period you are working on the problem and before it's time to work on coitus. You also should not engage in any other sexual activity together besides the exercises until he has developed reasonably good control. It's fine, though, to put aside time that your partner just spends pleasuring you.

Penile Touch Desensitization and Sensitization

EXERCISE 1: Solo Stop-Start

The first of these exercises is done by the man on his own. If done correctly, it will help reduce his anxiety and increase his focus as well as increase his confidence that he can have control.

Lasting longer also means more intense orgasms, so mastering this exercise provides motivation for wanting to last longer with a partner.

The man should begin by masturbating as he usually does but without fantasy or any other mental stimulation. The idea is for him to stay focused on the physical sensations. If he isn't able to sustain an erection without fantasy, he can move back and forth between fantasy and sensate focus, keeping in mind that the more focused he is physically, the more progress he will make.

Once he is able to get an erection by focusing on the good sexual sensations he is experiencing, he's ready to begin monitoring his level of arousal as he moves toward orgasm. Ask him to imagine arousal on a scale of zero to ten, with zero being no arousal and ten being orgasm. Somewhere between eight and nine he will reach the point of ejaculatory inevitability. Once he reaches that point, there is absolutely nothing he can do to stop himself from coming. He needs to learn to slow the movement toward orgasm earlier, somewhere between six and seven on the arousal scale.

When he thinks that he is close to having an orgasm, he should stop stimulating himself and breathe deeply until the strong urge to ejaculate goes away. If this takes more than fifteen or twenty seconds, he needs to stop earlier. He should then rearouse himself, stopping again when he feels he is getting close, but not too close, to orgasm. He should repeat this sequence three times. Then, the fourth time, he can bring himself to a climax.

If he's having a lot of trouble getting aroused to the point of orgasm without fantasy, he should try going back and forth between fantasy and a more direct focus on the physical sensations. Again, the more time he is able to spend getting in touch with the physical feelings associated with arousal, the better his progress will be.

If he has been masturbating by rubbing against a mattress or pillow, he needs to start using his hand. The best way to make this transition is to spend a few weeks exploring the sensations from manual stimulation without expecting to become very aroused. Eventually, he will become accustomed to using his hand and can go on to practicing the stop-start exercise. It is imperative, however, that he give up rubbing as a way of masturbating. It's much more difficult to discern and modify levels of arousal with this form of self-stimulation. That makes it counterproductive to developing good ejaculatory control.

He should be able to last ten to fifteen minutes by himself before moving on to practicing with you. If the exercise takes only a few minutes, he is probably stimulating himself too close to the point of no return before stopping.

If he is able to do the exercise successfully but doesn't find it pleasurable, he is completely focused on the pleasure of orgasm, ignoring the pleasure of arousal. As a result, he often has little motivation to develop control other than to please his partner. "I like the feeling of orgasm better than anything else," a twenty-six-year-old banking assistant told me. "All the sensual stuff feels okay, but orgasm is really what it's all about." This man never developed good ejaculatory control because a large part of him was not really interested in prolonging his orgasm.

EXERCISE 2: Head-to-Toe Desensitization with Penile Touch

Once your partner has developed some control on his own, you and he can begin working together. This exercise is designed to help a man with PE relax when being touched by a partner as well as to break what is often almost a reflexive overresponse to mild genital stimulation.

This exercise supports many of the exercises that follow, so doing it successfully is important. Begin with your partner lying down and you sitting up. Position yourself comfortably, and ask your partner to close his eyes and relax; use a blindfold if it helps. Start by touching him in a passive, nonsexual way—almost a patting motion—and then move to a touch that is more tender and sensual. Go very slowly and methodically. If he feels nervous, distracted, or aroused, he should let you know. When this happens, stop moving your hand and let it rest where it is. Instruct him to breathe deeply while bringing a relaxing image to mind. If he has trouble thinking of a relaxing scene, he can just think the word "calm." Once his anxiety subsides, you can go back to touching him.

As you continue, your touch should become more sexual and geared toward arousing him. However, the goal of this exercise is not for you or your partner to have an orgasm, so you should alternate between a sexual and sensual touch. Once again, if your partner becomes nervous, distracted, or overly aroused, stop stimulating him and have him breathe deeply and bring a calming image to mind. Repeat this exercise until he can enjoy having his penis touched without experiencing anxiety or a lot of arousal.

EXERCISE 3: Stop-Start with a Partner

STEP A: Alternate Touching

Begin by relaxing together with either the yoga or synchronized breathing. Then take turns touching each other in a sensual way. The reason it's better to start with alternate touching is that it will be easier for your partner to focus. Do not let him stimulate you to orgasm because it may overly excite him. Rather, after he has caressed you pleasingly for a while, ask him to be passive, and begin touching him in a gentle, increasingly sexual way. After a while begin stimulating his penis with your hands until he has a full erection.

When he begins to feel close but not too close to orgasm, he should tell you to stop. Wait about twenty seconds for his arousal to dissipate. Depending on his age, he may lose some of his erection. Once the strong urge to ejaculate has eased, stimulate him again to the point where he tells you he's about to come and then stop. Do the stop-start three times. After the fourth arousal, stimulate him to an orgasm.

After he has mastered this exercise with manual stimulation, you can alternate with your mouth, lips, and tongue if you enjoy oral sex. Most men will appreciate your efforts.

You know he is making progress when he enjoys the experience and is able to last as long or almost as long with you as by himself.

If he ejaculates very quickly or can last only a very short time between stops, a number of things may be happening. First, he may have become overly aroused from having touched you. If this is the case, move much more slowly and have him verbalize what he is feeling as he is touching you.

Another possibility is that he is very anxious about whether or not he is going to have good control. As a result, he can't really focus on what he is feeling in his body and is losing control. This type of premature ejaculation is much more related to nervousness than to actual arousal. If this happens, begin by letting your hand rest passively on his penis, while he breathes deeply and relaxes. Then proceed with the exercise very slowly, making sure to stop and relax if his anxiety starts to get the best of him.

If he does not get an erection or have an orgasm, he is probably trying to control his arousal by thinking of the exercise in a tasklike way. As a result, he may not be aroused at all. It is very important that you do not construe his inability to get hard or his *not* having an orgasm as a sign that the problem is getting better. Developing control is about having the ability, within reason, to have an orgasm if and when he wants to. If your partner is overcontrolling, you need to reinforce the idea that it is better for him to come quickly while practicing the exercises, at least at first, then to try to overcontrol his responses. If, however, he continues to struggle, then you should do exercises for erection problems before continuing.

Once you have done Step A successfully two or three times, you are ready to move on to the next step.

STEP B: Stop-Start with Mutual Touching

This exercise uses the same basic stop-start technique, except that rather than start with alternate touching, the two of you engage in mutual foreplay. This will obviously be more exciting for you and your partner, so it is important that even before you get to a lot of genital touching, you slow the pace if you think he is rushing ahead.

You will know that he's making progress if he exhibits the same control as he did during the stop-start exercises with alternate touching. If his arousal skyrockets, he may be plugging into your excitement as if it were his own. In order to correct this, the mutual sex play should move along much more slowly. Remind him to focus on what he is feeling in his body and to pay less attention to what is going on in yours.

STEP C: Stop-Slow with Alternating Passivity

Once your partner can control his ejaculation by stopping, he is ready to monitor himself by slowing down. It's best to start with your partner being passive so he can really focus. Stimulate him until he becomes a little more than moderately aroused, at which point he should instruct you to slow down. Initially you might find that he needs to slow down again soon after the first slowdown. What that tells you is that he is allowing himself to become too aroused before asking you to slow the pace. By relaxing and keying into his level of arousal, he will become increasingly adept at being able to sustain a moderately high level of arousal without coming too quickly.

STEP D: Stop-Slow with Mutual Touching

This step is an advanced version of the stop-slow with passivity because you will be touching each other simultaneously. That means he will be more excited. Don't be discouraged if your partner has to slow down early and often in order to maintain control. In time he will develop the ability to receive increasing amounts of stimulation without becoming excessively excited.

Penetration Desensitization

It is not uncommon for a premature ejaculator who has reached this point in treatment to say, "This is all fine, but what's going to happen when I actually have sex?" A man like this views intercourse and having sex as equivalent, one of the reasons that he has so much trouble with penetration to begin with. Therefore, don't be surprised if it takes him a lot longer to master the following advanced exercises, even if he has made excellent progress up to this point.

Penetration desensitization exercises are intended to help a man develop greater ejaculatory control with penetration at that critical point in sex that men with sexual problems—especially PE—have so much difficulty with. First, a man needs to recognize that the mental, not the physical, aspect of intercourse is causing his inability to have control. If you could measure the physical sensations of intercourse or monitor sensations on some sort of sexual seismograph, you would find no significant difference between penetration and other forms of stimulation. If anything, penetration probably is less physically stimulating than masturbating. Getting a man to understand this intellectually is one thing; getting him to develop better control by responding to the actual physical sensation of penetration and intercourse takes time and patience. The following exercises can help.

EXERCISE 1: Penetration Desensitization in the Female Superior Position

STEP A: Penis near the Vagina

This exercise helps desensitize a man to what is often an automatic increase in arousal simply by virtue of being near the vagina. The anticipation of intercourse can be enough to get his arousal barreling out of control.

Begin with either your partner passively receiving while you stimulate him or with you both engaging in mutual arousal—whichever he finds more relaxing and less distracting. If you notice that it is harder for him to concentrate on his own sensations when he touches you, he should just receive. If touching you helps him focus and override his anxiety, then mutuality is the better choice.

After stimulating him for a brief period of time, get on top and gently rub the length of his penis against the lips of your vagina. It does not matter if he has an erection at this point or not. If he feels as if he is becoming overly aroused after a while, he should return to deep breathing and relaxing imagery until the excitement level subsides. Then you can begin again. As you continue stimulating him, spread the lips of your vagina, and move his penis around inside the lips, but not inside your vagina. Once again you need to stop and have him refocus on what he is actually feeling in his penis if he gets too close to orgasm. Repeat the stop-start sequence three times, and then, the fourth time, bring him to orgasm on the inner lips of your vagina.

If he loses his erection during the exercise, he is mentally overcontrolling. That is, he is thinking about work or dirty laundry or something else totally unrelated to what he's doing in a vain attempt to prevent himself from becoming overly aroused. Remind him that trying to control his arousal in this way does not cure PE and can cause other problems.

You are ready to move on to the next step, once he is able to have a relaxed attitude about his penis being near your vagina.

STEP B: Insertion with No Movement

Mastering this step will demonstrate to a premature ejaculator that the physical sensations of penetration are not so sensational as to immediately catapult him to orgasm.

After an extended period of foreplay, sit astride your partner, take his penis in your hand, and insert it slowly, a little bit at a time. Once it is fully inserted, sit quietly for a few seconds. Then slowly ease his penis out of your vagina and go back to manual stimulation. Repeat this sequence of penetration, followed by manual stimulation, three or four times. He can then have an orgasm, but not inside you.

If he feels he is about to come the minute he puts it in or if he actually does come, you may have initiated penetration when he was too aroused. On a scale of one to ten, his arousal should be no more than a five or six. He also needs to be very relaxed before mastering this step. If he is tensing up right before insertion, have him breathe deeply until his anxiety subsides. Asking your partner to verbalize what he is feeling can be helpful. Once he realizes that it is the idea of penetration, not the actual sensation associated with penetration, that is knocking his socks off, his control will become much better.

Continue this exercise until penetrating your vagina does not cause his arousal to blow through the roof.

STEP C: Full Penetration with Movement

When penetration with no movement ceases to be a problem, you are ready to move on to being more active during coitus.

Begin with a period of slow, mutual foreplay. Let your partner know when you're wet enough. After that it is his responsibility to let you know when to initiate intercourse. He should be moderately aroused but not so turned on that he is close to the point of orgasm.

After penetration, have your partner place his hands on your hips so he can guide your movements. He should slow you down or have you stop if he feels close to coming. Wait until his arousal dissipates, and begin again.

If he seems to be doing fine but his arousal suddenly goes berserk, anxiety is getting the best of him. If this is a problem, your partner needs to be aware of when he is becoming tense and to stop the moment he becomes nervous. Once a man starts worrying about losing control, his control from that point on is going to be tenuous. Remind him that it is better to slow things down too early than too late.

If, after many attempts, he still seems to ejaculate with little warning, he may be suffering from an intense dread of a woman's disapproval. Your patience and positive attitude may be enough to help him through this. At the same time, if either of you is starting to feel extremely frustrated, it may be advisable to seek professional help.

Repeat this step until he feels increasingly confident that he can control the timing of his orgasm in this position. Remember, no one is perfect. Progress is what is important.

EXERCISE 2: Experimenting with Different Positions

A lot of men (and women) have the idea that once a man has developed decent control with a woman on top, he is home free. Often this is not the case, however. This fact of life can lead to a great deal of frustration, especially in light of the anxious, goal-oriented personalities that men with PE often have.

"I feel like I'm back to square one," a thirty-one-year-old man told me. Gil had made great progress up to this point but had come within thirty seconds after he penetrated his partner in the male superior position. Certain positions—male superior and rear entry in particular—are more physically stimulating to a lot of men. There are also more things that a man needs to focus on in these positions, such as where his hands go or if his arms are getting tired. These can distract him from focusing on the physical sensations in his body, making good control harder to come by.

Unless you're happy to have sex in only one position, there are a number of things you can do to foster better control in different positions. First, rehearse each position before you actually use it during sex. Figure out where all the hands, arms, and legs go or whether you need a pillow under your hips. Most important, figure out the best way for him to get his penis in. That way he won't have to hunt and peck later on.

It is a good idea, with every new position, to go through the steps of slow insertion with no movement followed by penetration with limited movement before you attempt intercourse with full movement. It might also be easier for you to start with a position such as side by side, either with both of you face-to-face or with your back to his. This position is less physically stressful than many others and can make it easier for your partner to focus on control.

If at any point his arousal seems to spiral quickly out of control, it probably means that he is speeding up too fast. Over time he will develop greater knowledge of how fast or slow he should go in order to maintain maximum control.

Finally, a technique called grinding can be very useful in positions where your partner is doing most of the moving.

EXERCISE 3: Grinding

This is a great alternative to thrusting during intercourse because it is pleasurable to a woman and less arousing to a man.

Grinding involves moving the body in a circular, as opposed to a back-and-forth, motion. First practice this motion with you on top. Be sure to roll your hips, rather than simply rub back and forth. After you show him how, ask him to practice by himself and then with you during sex. After arousing, he can slowly penetrate in the male superior position. He should keep his penis deep inside and move slowly in a circular fashion. As always, he should stop or slow down when he feels he's becoming too aroused.

Overall he should be able to maintain better control with this motion than by thrusting. If he doesn't or seems to be flopping around, he just hasn't gotten the movement right yet. Go back to rehearsing. Eventually he'll get the hang of it.

A man with PE should ultimately be able to control his orgasm in various positions. That does not mean that his control will be equally good in all positions, however. Each man has certain positions that are more stimulating and bring him to the point of no return faster than others.

It's important to keep in mind that there is no way that a man will not lose control some of the time. As time goes on, these instances will decrease. But if either of you is expecting perfection, you're headed for disappointment.

If nothing still seems to work and his PE doesn't seem to be significantly better, or there are times when he seems to have control while at other times he seems to be back at square one, he may not really want to have control. Remember, control is a choice. If a man chooses to ignore the necessary steps for developing control—to focus on the physical sensations and to avoid rushing ahead—he is making a conscious decision not to have control. That is his right, of course. But being unwilling to live with that choice is your right.

EXERCISES FOR ERECTION PROBLEMS

Helping a man overcome an erection problem is often more difficult than resolving PE because erection difficulties tend to create more performance pressure and anxiety. The good news is that with patience and a positive outlook, the likelihood of success is excellent.

You should not rush through the exercises. You should also avoid the temptation to have intercourse even if your partner swears up and down that he's ready. The exercises should be done in sequence. The only other permissible sexual contact while you're practicing is to have your partner sexually pleasure you.

The partner exercise should be practiced three times a week, and the masturbation once or twice a week. Since erections are so temperamental, you need to be flexible. If a man is not in the mood for sex, wait a day or so until he is. Obviously he's resisting if he often seems to find a reason not to practice. The two of you should deal with this immediately and get back on track.

Penile Touch Desensitization and Sensitization

These exercises help a man learn to focus on the sensations in his body when his penis is being touched, without worrying about whether or not he gets an erection.

The first message that a man with an erection problem needs to get through his head is that an erection lost does not mean an erection gone forever. This is crucial. It is common for a man to quit as soon as he begins losing his erection or feels it wavering. Once he discovers that he can recover from a decline in arousal during sex, his sensitivity to every change in his level of arousal will decrease dramatically, and with it, his overall performance anxiety.

EXERCISE 1: Solo Stop-Start

This first exercise is to be done by your partner alone. Mastering this exercise will give him the confidence that his body can and will respond if he is relaxed and stimulated properly.

He should pick a time when he can relax. Lying on his back and using his hand, he can begin stimulating himself in an inquisitive, exploratory way, almost as if he were learning about what he enjoys for the first time. Ask him to look for a particular spot that feels especially good when he touches himself or a particular stroke he enjoys.

He should arouse himself slowly *without fantasizing or looking at sexually explicit pictures or reading erotic material.* At first he may find it difficult to get an erection without additional mental stimulation. Many men with erection problems have become dependent on fantasy for sexual excitement. Since the fear of not getting an erection is so powerful, a man's natural inclination will be to use the method he has come to rely on. If fantasies do creep into his mind, he can refocus by saying to himself, "Stop thinking about this sexy fantasy, and go back to focusing on what you are feeling in your body right now."

Even if he can get an erection, it will probably take him longer to become aroused without fantasy. He may not even get a full erection the first few times he tries. He needs to be persistent and have faith. If he's determined to overcome the problem, he will.

If he continues to struggle, suggest that he use fantasy to get started and then go back to focusing on the pleasure of the physical sensations. Eventually, as he becomes more confident about his erection, he will feel less threatened by an inability to arouse immediately.

When he begins to feel that he is nearing orgasm, he should stop stimulating himself and wait for most of his erection to subside. During this time instruct him to breathe deeply and relax. Then he should begin rearousing himself to the point where he is fairly close to orgasm. Once again he should stop and wait for his erection to subside. Then he should restimulate himself, and this time, if he wishes, he can use sexual fantasy and have an orgasm.

You can tell he's making progress when he is able to regain his erection after losing it and when he begins to trust that if his body is stimulated properly, it will respond consistently.

If, after many attempts, his equipment still fails to respond, or he gets an erection but never feels close to orgasm, he should try using fantasy. Whether it's performance anxiety about his erections or lack of sensate awareness that's doing him in, going too long without success will only create more anxiety. Have him do the exercise, incorporating fantasies or other sexual imagery, and stop when he gets an erection rather than when he's close to coming. Although not ideal, this will at least begin giving him the confidence that he can gain an erection, lose it, and regain it. With some success under his belt, he can then start to wean himself off fantasy and get focused on the pleasurable physical sensation of sex.

EXERCISE 2: Head-to-Toe Desensitization with Penile Touch

One of the most important things that a man with an erection problem needs to learn is that it's okay for him not to get hard the instant a woman touches his penis. A lot of men believe that they should automatically get it up just being around a naked woman, so when a man's penis doesn't spring to attention when he is fondled, his angst can be enormous.

The purpose of this exercise is to help a man become comfortable with having his penis caressed without getting an erection. This exercise supports many of the exercises that follow, so doing it successfully is important. Begin with your partner lying on his stomach and you sitting up. Position yourself comfortably, and ask your partner to close his eyes and relax; use a blindfold if it helps. Start by touching him in a passive, nonsexual way—almost a patting motion—and then move to a touch that is more tender and sensual. Go very slowly and methodically. If he feels nervous, distracted, or aroused, he should let you know, and you should stop moving your hand and let it rest where it is. Instruct him to breathe deeply while bringing a relaxing image to mind. If he has trouble thinking of a relaxing scene, he can just think the word "calm."

Once his anxiety subsides, you can begin playfully stroking his penis. Have fun. Try different touches. Feel how soft the skin is. The goal is not to arouse him but to teach him to enjoy the feeling of having his nonerect penis touched.

If he does become aroused or feels pressured to have an erection, stop stimulating him and have him breathe deeply, again bringing a calming image to mind. Repeat this exercise until he can enjoy having his penis touched without experiencing arousal or anxiety.

Don't be surprised if at first he has trouble remaining passive. Although you may think that most men enjoy nothing better than being "done to," many men with erection problems have a hard time just receiving pleasure. The idea of lying back with an exposed flaccid penis can make a man feel very vulnerable. He may also feel self-conscious if he thinks his penis is not big enough.

Whatever the case, getting a man comfortable with being touched while in a nonaroused state is an important step in solving his problem. Keep practicing until the two of you have accomplished this goal.

EXERCISE 3: Stop-Start with a Partner

STEP A: Male Is Passive

After your partner is able to relax and focus on the sensations with a flaccid penis, the next step is for him to learn to stay relaxed while he is being sexually stimulated. The stated goal is not for him to have an erection but to stay in tune with the sensations he's feeling as you stroke his penis. If he does that, and you're touching him in a way that he enjoys, he will inevitably get an erection.

Begin with synchronized breathing, followed by foreplay. Have your partner lie on his back or side, and stimulate him until his erection is firm. Then stop the stimulation, and wait for his erection to subside. You can continue to touch him in a less sexual way as long as you allow his erection to subside. Then rearouse him, and help him have an orgasm.

The first few times that you do this exercise, stop only once. After he is comfortable doing this, repeat the exercise, stopping the stimulation and rearousing him twice before bringing him to orgasm.

If he does not get an erection, or if his erection fluctuates wildly, he is worrying about his performance. When this happens, stop the exercise and help him relax and regain focus on the physical sensations in his body. Then start again. Ignoring the worry and the self-monitoring that accompanies it or trying to push through it does not work. The only consistent way to get rid of his anxiety is to stop each and every time he begins to monitor himself and to have him relax, and then return to sensate focus.

Also, make sure that you are touching him in a pleasurable way. Encourage him to instruct and guide you during the exercise. Even though you may generally have a good understanding of what he enjoys, only he can know what he would like at a particular moment.

If he loses his erection when you stop stimulating him and rearouses fairly easily when you start touching him again, you can go to the next step.

STEP B: Stop-Start with Mutual Foreplay

This exercise is exactly the same as the stop-start exercise with passivity except that this time your partner can stimulate you as you are touching him. He should be reminded that most of his arousal should come from your touching him. It is perfectly natural for him *not* to have an erection simply from caressing and arousing you. Follow the basic stop-start instructions, going through the sequence at least three times. It's fine for both of you to have an orgasm.

Most men find the stop-start exercise with mutual touching easier than when they are passive. That's because touching you provides an added sexual charge. It also gives a man something else to think about besides the status of his erection.

If you notice that he is having a problem sustaining an erection, however, he may be overly focused on how aroused you are (or aren't). Repeat the exercise with the understanding that he should be touching you for his pleasure, not yours. If he becomes distracted by how good a job he's doing pleasing you, he should stop and refocus. Let him know if you would like to have an orgasm, but it's perfectly fine for him to help you come after he does.

If he still continues to lose his erection with mutual stimulation, you may be dealing with a desire disorder rather than an erection problem. The exercises in the following chapter will be of value, if that is the case.

Penetration Desensitization

Let's face it. As uptight as a man may be about foreplay, the real anxiety is intercourse. There is a profound fear of intercourse among men with every type of disorder because it is viewed as the ultimate goal, the real test.

Therefore, it should come as no surprise that desensitizing a man to the fear of losing his erection at the point of or during intercourse is a major part of successfully resolving his sexual difficulties.

EXERCISE 1: Condom Training

Understandably, in the minds of a lot of men, a condom signals intercourse. Therefore, by learning to deal nonchalantly with a condom, a man will automatically reduce the anxiety associated with intercourse. Even if the two of you do not use a condom regularly, doing this exercise can be of enormous benefit.

Unwrap a bunch of condoms of your choice, and leave them readily available on the bed. You and your partner can fondle each other simultaneously, or he can remain passive, whichever he prefers. When he has a semierection, put on a condom and practice the stop-start partner exercise for erection problems. If he loses his erection either before or after the condom is on, stop, have him breathe deeply and relax, and then restimulate him. Do this until he can successfully practice the stop-start exercise with a condom.

He may complain at first that he cannot feel anything with "this rubber glove on my cock," as one patient described it. This is usually a cover-up for his performance anxiety about intercourse. Although it is true that there is a loss of sensation with a condom, I have not had one patient who has not been able to get used to a condom with some practice.

If he continues to resist or to withdraw, suggest that he first try to use a condom while masturbating. Once he is comfortably using a condom by himself, it will become less of a problem with a partner.

EXERCISE 2: Penetration Desensitization in the Female Superior Position

The next series of exercises employs a step-by-step approach to helping a man become comfortable first with penetration and ultimately with intercourse. Each step is intentionally a baby step forward. It's a lot better for a man's ego to have success taking a small step than to fail taking a big one.

You should not be surprised if each step needs to be done a number of times. The anxiety a man has built up around intercourse can be very intense and takes time to overcome. A positive attitude on your part is critical. If you become worried, it will only exacerbate his own exaggerated concern.

STEP A: Penis near the Vagina

This exercise reduces the enormous performance anxiety that a man with erection problems experiences when he's anywhere near the vagina.

Begin with either your partner passively receiving while you stimulate him or engage in mutual arousal—whichever he finds more relaxing and less distracting. If you notice that it is harder for him to concentrate on his own sensations when he touches you, he should just receive. If being more involved helps him focus and override his anxiety, then mutuality is the best choice.

After stimulating him for a brief period of time, get on top of him, and gently rub the length of his penis against the lips of your vagina. It does not matter if he has an erection or not. If he becomes overly anxious or aroused, he should return to deep breathing until the level of excitement subsides; then you can begin again. Repeat this sequence a number of times. As you continue stimulating him, spread the lips of your vagina and move his penis around inside the lips but not inside your vagina. Once again, if he gets too close to orgasm, stop and have him refocus on what he is actually feeling in his penis. Repeat the stop-start sequence three times, and then, the fourth time, bring him to orgasm on the inner lips of your vagina.

If he loses his erection every time his penis gets near your vagina, his anxiety is getting the best of him. Talk to him about exactly what is going on in his mind as you place his penis near your genitals. He should be focus only on the good sensations of your wet inner lips. To make progress, he has to stop thinking and start feeling what is happening in his body. Repeat the exercise using a combination of deep breathing and relaxing imagery. If he still is losing his erection, suggest that he use some fantasy for the time being to circumvent his anxiety and self-monitoring.

If he is not successful after two or three attempts, stop the exercises completely and seek professional help. Either the extent of his performance anxiety is more than you can deal with alone, or the cause of his problem is more serious than you think.

STEP B: Getting Used to Insertion

After doing the above exercise successfully several times, move on to intercourse. This step is intended to help a man who's terrified of intercourse to begin viewing it as a continuation of foreplay rather than as a completely different experience.

You should make sure you are well lubricated before beginning this exercise. You will be inserting your partner's penis in his time frame, not yours. Using an artificial lubricant such as K-Y jelly or Albolene will ensure that insertion goes smoothly.

Begin with synchronized breathing followed by mutual stimulation. Then have your partner lie on his back as you sit astride him. Stimulate him until he has an erection. Move his penis sensually around the mouth of your vagina. Then take his penis in your hand, and insert it *very* slowly, a little bit at a time. Once it is fully inserted, get off your partner, and go back to manual stimulation. Repeat the sequence of penetration followed by manual stimulation three times, and then bring him to an orgasm manually.

Do the exercise until there is little or no fluctuation in his erection when he enters you.

STEP C: Full Penetration in Female Superior

After developing confidence that he can sustain an erection with penetration, the next step is to try the same basic procedure with movement—otherwise known as intercourse.

Begin with a long period of slow, mutual foreplay. If you need a lubricant, use one. Let your partner know that it is his responsibility to tell you when he is ready for intercourse. He should be aroused but not close to coming.

After penetration, have your partner place his hands on your hips so that he can guide your movements. He should slow you down or have you stop if he begins to lose his erection or becomes anxious that he might lose his erection.

If his erection goes away, get off him, and have him breathe deeply and relax until he can refocus. Then, after stimulating him manually or orally to an erection, begin again.

Repeat this until he feels increasingly confident that he can sustain an erection in this position.

There are a number of things that you can do if he continues to lose his erection during intercourse. First, try to figure out if there is a pattern to when he loses his arousal. You might find that he loses sensation if you move too quickly, for example. Another possibility is that your partner may be worried that he'll come too fast. This is particularly true if he has a history of premature ejaculation. Let him know that control is not the issue; you can deal with that problem later, when he has more confidence in his erection.

If he is still having erection problems, then do the above exercise with shorter bouts of penetration. Allow him to lose his erection on purpose when you get off him, rearouse him manually, and then go for another short bout of intercourse. This on and off sequence, coupled with giving a man permission to lose his erection, can be very effective.

Problems that continue to persist require professional intervention.

EXERCISE 3: Experimenting with Different Positions

Once your partner is comfortable in intercourse with you on top, you can try other positions. This may not be as easy as it appears. A lot of men have a great deal of anxiety about going from one position to another because they are afraid they will lose their erections during the switches in position. Therefore, it's a good idea for you at first to continue stimulating him manually or for him to continue stimulating himself as he moves from one position to the next. Plan on working on each position numerous times so that the two of you can determine the ones you like best.

Success for a man with an erection problem means he does not become overly anxious in the process of changing positions and is able to maintain an erection in different positions. Keep in mind he may find certain positions more stimulating than others. Rather than insist that he be able to make love in any one way, you should aim to find a few positions that the two of you agree are fun and exciting.

One caveat here: Many men with erection problems have trouble adjusting to being on top. Most often this happens because they have not found a way to be physically comfortable in this position. This may sound funny, but it's true. There are a lot of men who can't seem to figure out how to balance their bodies or where to place their arms. Men who are not in good shape physically complain that this position (and sometimes others that also require more activity) is too strenuous.

It might be helpful to rehearse various positions. That way your partner can become increasingly comfortable with what to do with all his body parts without having to worry about his control or erection. If exhaustion is the issue, it's time he got into aerobics or weight lifting.

If he continues to lose his erection except when you are on top, he probably has extreme performance anxiety. Since he has to work to move into most other positions, the five seconds he has to do without stimulation may be sending him into a panic. To help ease the transition, it can be useful for you or him to continue stimulating his penis as he gets into position.

Another reason that a man may have problems with being on top is that he doesn't know how to find the vaginal opening. Of course, he will never tell you this. "I would feel ridiculous asking her, 'Where in the hell does this thing go anyway?'" is the way one man put it. Fortunately this problem is easy to solve. Stop leaving the guesswork to him, and guide him in. Instructing him how to find the opening on his own when there is no sexual activity can also be very helpful.

If the problem persists, there may be a deeper psychological component at work. Being on top is a power position for a man or a woman. The fear of being on top can reflect an underlying discomfort with being sexually aggressive. If you suspect something like this is the case, it is advisable that you seek professional help.

PHARMACEUTICALS—AIDS TO AROUSAL

If, after completing the exercises, your partner still has trouble either getting or sustaining an erection, he needs professional assistance. If he has not already seen a urologist and is unable to get or sustain an erection with masturbation, a visit to a physician is the first step. At the very least a doctor should check a man's testosterone level and his penile pulse and give him an at-home device to test for nocturnal erections. In some cases, more extensive testing may be warranted. Be wary of any doctor who prescribes any sort of invasive measure without in-depth testing.

Even if the tests are negative, the problem may still be organic in nature. It is likely, however, that the physical part of his problem is not very significant.

If there is no detectable organic problem and your partner is still not having any success with the exercises, there are a few other things worth trying. The first and least invasive technique is to use sexual fantasy to assist in his arousal. In cases of extreme performance anxiety, incorporating fantasy together with sexually explicit films and books can be very helpful in overriding nervousness. Fantasy can also increase a man's level of arousal and help him sustain a shaky erection when he might otherwise lose it.

Even when a man's problem is all in his head, he can reach a point of such frustration and fear of failure that medical intervention may be warranted. For most men, the treatment of choice will be Viagra. Viagra works by increasing the blood flow to the penis. Depending on the severity of the problem, a man may take from 25 to 100 milligrams one hour before he plans to engage in sexual activity. Viagra will not produce an automatic erection. A man will need direct stimulation for Viagra to work.

Viagra can have a lot of benefits. Obviously, for the man who has an organic problem, it can help him do what his body can't do alone. For the man whose problem is psychological, the effects can be profound. There is no better boost for getting erections than having one. By being able to get and consistently keep an erection, a man will feel less anxious about his erections. The result is that in time he may feel more and more turned on and less and less worried, and eventually he may not even need Viagra. Clearly, a relaxed and focused mind has the power to override a body that is not in perfect working order. If the problem is not organic, a man may eventually develop enough sexual confidence to begin weaning himself off Viagra.

Viagra also has some disadvantages. Some men experience undesirable side effects. The most common ones include a flushed feeling, headaches, palpitations, and a visual distortion where one sees blue. Also, Viagra may be psychologically habit forming. In rare cases, Viagra has been fatal.

At the very least, before embarking on a course of Viagra, a man should be warned that it does not work for everyone. I cannot tell you the disappointments and frustrations suffered by men who were led to believe that Viagra was a surefire way to resolve their erection problems, only to find that it was not.

I have seen Viagra fail in men with physical problems as well as in men who are young and have no physical problems whatsoever. That is why it is so important to combine Viagra with standard sex therapy. Most men develop a great deal of anxiety about their erections once they start having problems. So even if Viagra can help a man get an erection, he still needs to be relaxed and focused enough to be able to enjoy the pleasurable stimulation that he is receiving.

Even if Viagra does not work, a man need not despair. There are several other potential options. One is injection therapy. Under a urologist's supervision, a man is taught to inject himself with one or a combination of three drugs: prostaglandin, papaverine, or phentolamine. Don't worry, the needle is so small it does not hurt. The injection works by relaxing the muscles surrounding the arteries in the penis so that more blood can flow in. The medication needs to be kept refrigerated. The injections are administered shortly before sexual contact.

Injection therapy does have some disadvantages. A lot of men flinch when they hear about sticking a needle in their dicks. Another problem is that repeated injections can sometimes cause scarring.

For men who are needle shy, another possibility is an intraurethral suppository called Muse.™ Some men complain of burning, but others find it produces the desired result with no negative side effects.

Still other men find that the vacuum pump is the way to go. It is harmless and painless. It works by putting negative pressure on the penis, making it bigger and longer. A rubber ring at the base of the penis helps hold the erection. This device can be purchased through a urologist. It is not sexy, however. The two of you will have to get used to it, should you choose this route. If you think it might work, try it. If it produces the desired effect with no negative side effects, it may very well be the option for you.

As a last resort, a man may opt for a penile implant. Because of the advances in treating impotence, however, most doctors rarely feel it is advisable to take such a drastic measure.

WHEN HE'S STILL HAVING PROBLEMS

If, after completing the above exercises, you have seen little or no progress, you are bound to feel confused and frustrated. A number of things may be happening. If a man continues to lose his erection and you have ruled out an organically based problem, chances are that the problem is more deeply rooted than you think. It is possible that his inability to sustain an erection is a symptom of a desire disorder. If so, Viagra will be useless. If this is the case, you can try some of the exercises in the following chapter, but in all likelihood you or he will need to seek the assistance of a sex therapist.

10

Overcoming
Desire, Inhibition,
and Orgasm
Problems

How do you help someone whose desire for sex is inhibited by feelings that sex is shameful? What can you do for a man who is unable to have an orgasm with a partner? Is there any remedy for a man who functions perfectly well in every sexual relationship except the one to which he is emotionally committed?

These are the questions that typically arise in the treatment of men with inhibited desire and orgasm problems. The answers are not easy. Desire disorders and serious sexual inhibitions often represent long-standing issues related to sex, women, and intimacy. These underlying issues usually need to be addressed before the sexual problem can be resolved, and that can take a long time.

Another problem that makes treating a man with a serious desire disorder difficult is that he often does not get aroused by touching his partner in a sexual way. He may even feel some aversion. As a result, he may have a problem getting and keeping an erection. He also tends to have a less than satisfying touch to his partner and to view her as an obligation. This can make it hard for a woman to feel motivated to be sexual with him.

Finally, men with these disorders often have overly controlling personalities that make them resistant to owning up to their problems or to following therapeutic guidance. They also can be irascible, passive-aggressive, and generally difficult to be around.

The combination of these dynamics makes treating men with these problems a difficult and lengthy process, compared with men with premature ejaculation and most erection problems.

The treatment strategy for inhibited desire and orgasm problems is also very different from that of other sexual dysfunctions. In this chapter I shall share with you the strategies that are necessary conditions for change. I will discuss orgasm problems and inhibitions that are related to conflicts about sex and intimacy. A loss of desire that comes from a relationship on the rocks needs to be dealt with by relationship counseling, not sex therapy.

There are three steps to resolving problems of orgasm, desire, and inhibition:

Heightening his responsiveness to physical stimulation: Developing a strong sensate foundation for experiencing arousal with a woman is a cornerstone of getting over desire and orgasm problems. A man with a desire problem often does not get turned on mentally when he is with a woman sexually. An intense focus on pleasurable physical sensations provides another avenue for creating arousal, triggering a positive chain reaction. As he functions more successfully, he beings to develop a positive link between women and sex. Eventually, as he has more and more pleasure with a woman, that link becomes a bond.

Getting a man to this point is not easy. Men with desire problems and serious sexual inhibitions are like men with other sexual problems in that they are not in touch with what is going on in their bodies. A man with either of these problems is likely to have the additional problem of preferring the sensations he creates for himself when masturbating. Before you can deal with his problem directly, he needs to be weaned off the need for exactly the same stimulation he is accustomed to while masturbating. At the same time he has to teach his body to become more responsive to sensations that up until now he has not experienced as sexually arousing.

Using fantasy constructively: Even once he develops greater sensitivity to physical stimulation, it may not be enough to keep his juices flowing. Unlike a man with PE or impotence, who often overdoses on mental arousal during sex, an inhibited man blocks out the normal feelings of being turned on by the mental aspects of sex with a partner. Devoid of this basic component of arousal, teaching him to use fantasy is often a necessary adjunct to the primary focus on physical stimulation. Getting him to use fantasy to override his inhibitions when making love may take some convincing, however. Although the sexually inhibited man tends to get totally absorbed in fantasy when he masturbates, he may feel uncomfortable about using fantasy with a partner.

Striking the proper balance between focusing on fantasy and physical stimulation is the goal, but this can be a long, arduous process. If he becomes overly dependent on fantasizing while having sex, he will become completely dysfunctional when his fantasy does not click in at the appropriate moment.

Overcoming vaginal aversion: A man who is sexually inhibited also needs to work through the aversion to women's genitals that the overwhelming majority of these men have. He may never get to the point of enjoying using his tongue and lips to stimulate you, but if he cannot touch your wet throbbing parts with his fingers without feeling squeamish, he will never be able to enjoy sex fully. It is difficult to get a man to enjoy being inside a woman if he feels as if he is sticking his penis into something that he can barely tolerate touching or smelling.

VAGINAL-AVERSION DESENSITIZATION

Imagine that there is a food that for some reason has always made you feel queasy. (Soft-boiled eggs have that effect on me.) Now imagine that every time you make love, you have to touch, smell, and even eat that food. If you are grimacing, then you are starting to get a picture of how a man with a vaginal aversion feels.

Working to overcome an aversion to touching a woman's genitals takes time and practice, but it can be done. Getting a man comfortable with the smell and taste of a vagina is a lot more problematic and often may not be successful. So if receiving oral sex is high on your list of pleasurable activities, this man may not be the one for you.

Ground rules are very important. An aversion is usually symbolic of a strong fear. From the start your partner needs to feel that he is in control. He should do only as much as he can without feeling revulsion. If his negative reaction does not lessen or becomes greater after a number of tries, stop the exercises altogether. This response may suggest that the exercise are triggering unconscious memories of abuse. Any desensitization work from this point on should be done under the supervision of a therapist.

EXERCISE 1: Touch Desensitization

The first step is to help your partner become comfortable touching your genitals. If he is extremely aversive, you will want to start by having him rest his hand passively on the inside of your thigh, close to but not touching your vagina. One he's comfortable with this, he can move to the outside of your vagina. Relax. Try not to move. Talk about the best time you had together on vacation. If he begins to feel a negative response, he should remove his hand. Keep doing this until he can leave his hand on your vagina for a long time without having an adverse reaction.

Next, have your partner insert his finger inside your vagina and keep it there as long as he can without becoming uncomfortable. If he becomes really uncomfortable, he should remove his finger and do some deep breathing. If he becomes only a little anxious, he can leave his finger inside while breathing deeply and focusing on relaxing imagery. If he needs it, help him with the relaxing imagery. Stay relaxed yourself.

Repeat this process until he is able to explore your vagina with his finger without becoming queasy.

EXERCISE 2: Smell and Taste Desensitization

Neutralizing a man's aversion to the smell and taste of female vaginal secretions is usually more difficult and takes even more time than getting him comfortable touching it.

Since many men associate any body odor with being dirty, begin by taking a shower together. That way your partner will know that you are fresh and clean. When you are ready, ask him to put his finger slowly inside your vagina, to leave it in for a few seconds, and then slowly to bring his finger as close to his nose as he can tolerate. He should go slowly. Too much all at once is counterproductive. With each session he should try to bring his finger just a little closer to his nose.

The next step is for him to lick his finger and see what you taste like. Once again, stop if his anxiety skyrockets, and continue when it subsides. Repeat this until he can smell and taste you without reacting negatively.

The final step is for him to smell and taste you directly. Have him lie with his head between your legs or in the 69 position, whichever he finds more comfortable. At his own pace, have him lick your vagina, coming up for air if he becomes queasy. Do this for only very brief periods at first until his repulsion becomes neutralized.

If, after weeks of practicing, he starts to enjoy touching, smelling, or tasting you when you're making love, the prognosis for overcoming his desire or inhibition problem is excellent. On the other hand, if he can't even touch you unless you ask, he is still feeling repulsed. While a man with inhibitions will probably never consider your vagina one of your sweetest parts, if he can become at least neutral about it, he will want to touch it just to please you. If he continues to avoid touching you, he is still ill at ease. Keep working on the aversion exercises until he reaches a reasonable comfort zone.

Don't expect miracles. Although the overwhelming majority of men I have treated are able to resolve their aversions to the point that they no longer completely avoid a woman's genitals, it is very difficult to get a man who really dislikes oral sex to enjoy it. Remember, men with strong aversions usually have a lot of other sexual baggage. So if he is able to function relatively well as a lover and satisfy you with his hand or penis, consider yourself ahead of the game.

BECOMING COMFORTABLE USING
SEXUAL FANTASY

Throughout most of this book I have talked about how excessive fantasizing or mental arousal is an underlying cause of many sexual problems. So why am I suggesting that a man with desire problems or sexual inhibitions learn to fantasize? Because for a man with a desire disorder or orgasm problem, using sexual fantasy while having sex with a partner may be the only way to bolster his arousal and override his inhibitions.

Even though using fantasy during sex can be a great assistance, many men balk at the suggestion. And others who do fantasize often feel ashamed or guilty. A lot of men operate under the assumption that if a man has to fantasize when he's with a woman, either there is something wrong with him or he is not attracted to his partner. "Why isn't she enough to turn me on?" is a question he asks himself. Other men view fantasizing during sex as the mental equivalent of cheating. "My wife has gotten heavy and out of shape. So I feel guilty fantasizing about some twenty-three-year-old nymphet giving me oral sex," a man in his fifties who had a lifelong orgasm problem told me.

The strongest resistance to using fantasy, however, is embarrassment. A man with sexual inhibitions often has sadomasochistic, homosexual, or other fantasies that he thinks are perverted. When he fantasizes, even during masturbation, he is at war with himself. On the one hand, his fantasies turn him on. At the same time they disgust him. He may also fear that the more he fantasizes about something, the more likely he is to act on it. This prevents him from really enjoying himself and using fantasy to his benefit.

I explain to such a patient that fantasy is an integral part of sexual development. Trying to force-feed an "appropriate" fantasy in order to replace one you are uncomfortable with does not work. Worse yet, not using whatever fantasy spontaneously comes to mind interferes with sexual responsiveness.

Finally, fantasy is not the same as reality. A man who fantasizes about homosexual experiences is not necessarily gay any more than the woman who fantasizes about being raped actually wants to be raped. Also, not all fantasy needs to be self-generated. For some men, watching erotic movies or reading erotic books can have the same benefit as using their own self-created fantasies. The added advantage is that using erotic material can be very arousing and fun for you, too. The only drawback is that you and your partner may not be in sync on what turns you on. And since there is no right or wrong when it comes to fantasy, the sharing of arousing material will work only if the two of you have relatively similar tastes. Work to develop appreciation for one another's likes and dislikes, if that seems to help.

Once a man becomes comfortable using fantasy with his partner, amazing things begin to happen. I have worked with men who have had little or no sexual desire for years, who begin consistently to enjoy intercourse with their partners when they bring fantasy into their lovemaking. The combination of learning to focus on physical sensations and using fantasy to intensify that sensation is very powerful. Men who learn to use this combination will eventually overcome their problem.

Below are some exercises that can help.

EXERCISE 1: Exchanging Fantasies

Have you ever had a problem but felt too ashamed to talk to anyone about it because you thought that you were the only one with the problem? Do you remember the sense of relief you experienced when someone else shamefully told you he or she had the same problem? That is exactly how a man who is ashamed of his fantasies feels when his partner shares her fantasies with him.

Sharing your own sexual fantasies is the best and often the only way to get your partner to open up. It is only after you let him know that you will not judge him negatively for having fantasies and do not feel offended by them that he will feel open to sharing them and using them during sex.

EXERCISE 2: Penile Touch Desensitization Using Fantasy

This exercise is very similar to the penile touch desensitization exercise using relaxed imagery discussed in the last chapter. The difference is that when your partner becomes anxious or inhibited, rather than bring a calming image to mind, he should consciously focus on a sexual fantasy. Preparation is important. (Work on his fantasies with him if it helps.) He should have several to draw from before beginning the exercise.

Your partner should be nude and lying on his back with his eyes closed. Begin by touching his whole body in a sensual way with no emphasis on arousal. As he relaxes, fondle him in a way that is increasingly sexual.

At any point that he feels nervous, distracted, or bored, he should let you know. You should stop if he does not become aroused or if he grimaces or holds his breath. If this happens, stop caressing him and have him breathe deeply and relax. Once his tension subsides, tell him to keep up the deep breathing while focusing mentally on a very erotic scene.

Once his fantasy kicks in and his arousal returns, continue stimulating him. If he loses focus again, repeat the above procedure. Continue the exercise for fifteen or twenty minutes or until he has an orgasm, whichever comes first.

In time he should become increasingly adept using fantasies so that his arousal returns quickly if he loses it. You will be able to tell because there's a definite sense that he's into himself when he is fantasizing. Although this may be disconcerting at first, his detachment is a positive sign that he is able to tune you and his anxiety out while tuning his fantasy in.

EXERCISE 3: Having Him Touch You
While He Is Fantasizing

This exercise will help your partner get accustomed to being into his own head while being into your body.

Begin with synchronized breathing. Your partner should be behind you because he will feel more in control that way. As he relaxes, tell him to start fantasizing sexually. It is okay if he rubs his body against yours for some physical stimulation to get him going.

Once he is involved in his fantasy, instruct him to begin touching you slowly. Have him move his hand across your breast and thighs and ultimately touch your inner lips and clitoris. If he loses his fantasy or otherwise becomes distracted, he should stop. He can leave his hand resting where he was last touching while he does some deep breathing. When he is able to relax and recall the fantasy, he can start again. Repeat this exercise until he is able to touch you in an erotic way while focusing the sexual images in his mind.

If he continues to struggle with keeping his fantasy alive, chances are he is paying too much attention to pleasing you. Two things can help. First, you can tell him that for now he is to touch you without concern for how aroused you are becoming so that he can concentrate on his fantasy. Then, at another time, have him practice touching you solely for the purpose of pleasing you. Do this until he is comfortable. Then move on to doing the exercise with simultaneous touching.

If you notice over time that he gets excited while touching you, he's on his way to getting better. His pleasure in touching you will also make being with him sexually more fun for you.

EXERCISE 4: Weaning Him off Fantasy

Now that you've gotten your partner to feel comfortable incorporating fantasy into your sex life, you need to help him reduce his dependence on it. Although fantasy can go a long way toward boosting a man's level of arousal, if he is too dependent on fantasy, any noise or movement on your part can throw his arousal out of kilter. Men with this problem have told me that even the slightest sound on the part of their partners, such as a grunt or a moan, can distract them from their fantasies and turn them off. Unless you agree to be a mummy, this is obviously a problem because for a sexually healthy person, some form of noisemaking or other expression of sexual pleasure comes naturally.

The way around this dilemma is to wean him slowly from the need for silence while he is fantasizing. This will take time and patience. The best place to start is to have your partner communicate something he is enjoying during a sexual encounter. Suggest he make a slight noise. Or have him put his hand over yours when he is enjoying something that you are doing. Any verbal communication should be quick and to the point. Words like "faster," "slower," "now," "stop," and other simple utterances are about all that a man with this problem is going to be able to communicate for quite a long time.

The next step is for you slowly to introduce some sounds into your lovemaking. There needs to be an understanding on both your parts that your partner might lose his arousal at first. In time, though, he will become increasingly accustomed to hearing you while still being able to maintain focus on his fantasy. In addition, as he becomes less dependent on fantasy and responds more to direct physical stimulation, there will be a lot more room for you to communicate sexually with him while having sex without distracting him from the pleasurable sensations he is feeling.

EXPANDING HIS PHYSICAL RESPONSIVENESS

Like men with other sexual problems, a man who has an orgasm or a desire problem tends to be out of touch with his body. He also experiences the difficulty of being dependent on his own very specific form of mental and physical stimulation. Getting him in touch with what he is feeling in his body is not as simple as getting him to relax and focus on the pleasurable physical sensations because he is likely to feel very little unless the stimulation is exactly the same as that which he is accustomed to. First, a man has to become desensitized to his specific and often idiosyncratic needs. Then he needs to broaden the range of stimulation to which he can respond sexually.

The following exercises are important steps toward achieving those goals.

EXERCISE 1: Solo Stop-Start Using Fantasy

This exercise helps get a man more in touch with the arousal he is feeling in his body without depriving him of the mental stimulation he is used to. Ultimately the more he can get turned on from the pleasure of physical stimulation alone, the better off he will be.

The best way to get to this point is for him to begin by stimulating himself with his hand, jump-starting his arousal with the sexual fantasy of his choice. When he's feeling turned on, he can revert to concentrating on the physical sensations alone. If his arousal diminishes to the point that he feels he is going to lose his erection, he should bring in his fantasy again.

When he reaches the point at which he will have an orgasm if he continues, he should stop. After waiting fifteen seconds or so for the urge to dissipate, he should rearouse himself by alternating between fantasy and a focus on physical sensation.

Likewise, he should stop again when he's close to coming. After stopping and starting three times, he should masturbate to orgasm.

Patience is crucial. If his erection subsides every time he turns off the fantasy, he is convinced that he will never be able to arouse without fantasy or he is just being impatient. Giving him the proper frame of reference can be helpful. Explain that what he is doing is not something new. Rather, he is relearning something he used to be able to do a long time ago. Children learn to touch themselves not because they are mentally turned on but because the physical sensations associated with touching their genitals feel good. This understanding will give a man faith that learning to arouse without fantasy is not impossible. It will, however, take time, patience, and practice.

EXERCISE 2: Masturbation with Pelvic Thrusting

This exercise is a terrific way to begin weaning a man off the sensations that he is accustomed to during masturbation and getting him used to experiencing the sensations associated with intercourse.

In the same way that a man with a desire disorder or an inhibited orgasm problem is likely to have developed a strong dependence on fantasy, he is likely to have a similar dependence on very specific physical sensations that he provides for himself when he masturbates. In large part out of habit, he has come to associate a very limited range of sensations as sexually pleasurable. This exercise will help expand the range of sensations to which he can respond pleasurably.

He begins by stimulating himself in his usual fashion, using fantasy if he wants to. Then, when he reaches the point of ejaculatory inevitability and actually begins feeling his orgasm start, he should keep his hand still and thrust against it instead. The first few times he tries this he may experience his orgasm as little more than a blip as opposed to a bang. With practice, though, he will be able to have more intense orgasms with this thrusting motion.

At the outset he can alternate between thrusting and moving his hand. At first he will probably feel significantly less sensation when he thrusts than when he moves his hand. If he begins to lose his erection, he should go back to manually stimulating himself until he can regain a higher level of arousal. Then he can go back to thrusting.

If he repeatedly numbs out when he thrusts against his hand, he is probably obsessing about how much he is or is not feeling or thinking about how long it's taking or how futile the whole effort is. Whenever he feels this way, he needs to stop the action and breathe and relax until he can refocus. Then he can begin again.

The ultimate goal of the exercise is for him to feel as aroused with thrusting as with the manual motion.

EXERCISE 3: Having an Orgasm in Your Presence

A man who has a problem having an orgasm with a partner almost never has difficulty having one on his own unless he is taking some kind of medication that negatively affects the orgasm reflex. That's why the easiest way to get a man to reach orgasm with you is to have him masturbate when you are present.

Exactly how you should proceed depends on the man and the depth of his inhibition. One patient who suffered from this problem for most of his adult life found that the only way he felt comfortable enough was to have his wife sit on the other side of the room with blindfolds over her eyes and earplugs in her ears! Other men find that it is okay for their partners to lie on the bed with them but with their backs turned away. Still others find that the easiest route to success is for their partners to be stimulating themselves at the same time. This approach has a lot of benefits for dealing with this problem and for increasing sexual intimacy and closeness in general.

Once your partner has success bringing himself to orgasm in your presence, you should strive to increase gradually how close you lie together. Before going on to the next exercise, he should be able to climax comfortably while you hold him.

If orgasm defies him no matter how hard he tires, trying so hard is the problem. Whenever he gets frustrated, he should stop and relax. Trying to push through his frustration by working harder and harder to come will get nowhere. Relaxing, using fantasy, and focusing on the pleasurable physical sensations are the answer.

EXERCISE 4: Alternating Your Hand with His

The next step is to have your partner have an orgasm when you stimulate him.

He should stimulate himself until he begins having an orgasm. At this point put your hand over his. This will lay the basic foundation for associating his climax with your touch.

The next time your partner is aroused, take turns alternating between touching and squeezing his penis and then cupping it loosely with your hand moving up and down the shaft. Let him be in charge of telling you when he wants you to touch him and when he feels he wants to touch himself to maintain arousal. The first few times that you do this exercise, have him be the one to bring himself to orgasm with your hand over his. Once he is comfortable with this, you can work toward having him be able to reach his sexual peak with you stimulating him. You will have the most success with this exercise if you begin taking over the stimulation when he is very close to orgasm at first. Then you can gradually take over earlier and earlier during the session.

Eventually you will want to be able to bring your partner to orgasm manually exclusively with your stimulation. This will take time because your partner may not always be able to respond to your touch alone. If you are patient and do not expect 100 percent consistency, your partner will gradually become more responsive to you. Ask what he likes. Listen.

What if his arousal takes a nosedive each and every time you take over? Several things might be happening. You might not be touching him in a way that he finds particularly pleasurable. If he admits that this is true, ask him to show you where you're going wrong by having him put his hand over yours while you stimulate him. Eventually you should get the hang of how he likes it.

Another possible problem may be that he is monitoring himself. If this is the case, he will have to get to the point where he recognizes that he is not going to make progress unless he stops himself each time he wonders how he's doing. Sometimes it is only when a man becomes completely exasperated by his failure that this will sink in.

ASSOCIATING INTERCOURSE WITH PLEASURE AND ORGASM

Although a man with a long history of orgasm problems or a serious desire disorder will have come a long way after completing the above exercises, he may still have difficulty feeling the pleasure of sexual intercourse. There are a couple of reasons for this. He may have some deep-rooted or unconscious issues related to losing control or castration. More probable is the fact that a woman's vagina just doesn't feel the way his hand feels. While some men with inhibitions complain that vaginas are uncomfortably tight, most complain that they just don't have the same tight grip as their hand.

Either way, if a man does not experience intercourse as particularly pleasurable, he probably has the attitude that he will never find sexual satisfaction inside a woman. He may also have a tremendous fear that he won't be able to father a child. Overcoming this problem involves getting a man to associate intercourse with the pleasure of orgasm.

EXERCISE 1: Penetrating at the Point of Climax

Begin with either mutual foreplay or with your partner simply receiving stimulation, whichever you have determined to be more reliable. Then stimulate him with your hand or his hand or alternate between the two, to the point of orgasm. As he starts to come, put his penis inside you. Move until he stops coming. Have him rest inside you as long as he feels comfortable.

If he loses his orgasm when he penetrates, you are inserting him before he reaches the point of ejaculatory inevitability. This is the moment at which his orgasm is unstoppable. One observable sign is his testicles retracting inward toward his body. Make sure he has almost started to ejaculate before putting him inside. Don't be surprised if he cries in relief the first time he comes inside you.

Once you have done this successfully four or five times, you are ready to move on to the next step. This time incorporate short bouts of penetration in-between longer periods of manual or oral stimulation. Alternate back and forth between manual stimulation and penetration until your partner starts to come. Once again, initiate penetration at the point his climax begins.

If he cannot get to the point of orgasm once you begin incorporating penetration earlier than at the point of climax, he may be thinking too much about whether or not he will be able to come. If he loses concentration, have him breathe until he can refocus or get a fantasy going. Then stimulate him manually again until he is hard and ready to initiate intercourse again.

If he consistently loses his erection at the point of penetration, follow the penetration desensitization exercises for impotence in the last chapter, but have him incorporate fantasy. If after numerous attempts in different positions he is still losing his erection, you should seek professional help.

EXERCISE 2: Experimenting with Different Positions

One of the things that makes it difficult for a man with desire or orgasm problems to feel aroused is that he disregards sensations that he has not associated with high levels of arousal. He may tell you that he feels nothing during intercourse even though he has a rock-hard erection. What is really happening is that he is just not taking in the sensate messages he's receiving as pleasurable because it isn't a sexual feeling he is familiar with.

This exercise can be of tremendous value if done properly. Get yourselves aroused, and initiate penetration in any way the two of you choose. Move in different ways, and have him tell you which way you move feels best. Squeeze your vaginal muscles, and have him tell you what that feels like. Move your legs closer together or farther apart, and ask him to describe the difference. Hold his penis with your hand as he moves for additional stimulation. Experiment! Take your time. Make it fun.

Alert him before starting that he might lose his erection as he tries different things. That's okay! In the process of learning about what feels good, there will be times he will not feel that much. If and when this happens, simply rearouse him manually or orally, and initiate penetration again.

If he begins thrusting frantically, or grimaces, or numbs out, he is probably trying too hard. This desperation will only distract him from the feelings he needs to focus on in order to have a strong orgasm. What he needs to do when he starts losing sensation is to let you know, stop, and return to deep breathing, relaxing imagery, and his favorite sexual fantasy.

EXERCISE 3: Becoming More Responsive with Intercourse

In solving a sexual problem, you always want to take the path of least resistance. By focusing on the position your partner feels most comfortable with, you are going to have the best shot at success.

Either you or he can initiate intercourse in your favorite position. As always, he should incorporate fantasy when he needs to keep up his arousal. Also use any other strategy, such as holding his penis simultaneously or contracting your vaginal muscles, that increases his pleasure. If he loses sensation, revert to manual stimulation and try again. Continue until he is able to have an orgasm when he is thrusting inside you. Try different positions. Communicate. Be persistent.

WHAT NEXT?

Even if you seem to have made little progress after trying all these exercises, don't despair. He may still be able to overcome the problem with professional help. In some cases, a brief trial of Viagra may reduce the anxiety created by performance concerns. Usually, though, desire problems do not respond to pharmaceutical intervention. In this case, a certified sex therapist is your best bet. Finally, it is important for you to be honest, though, about whether you are willing to make the long-term commitment it is likely to take to resolve his problem. It is better to say no rather than to say yes but mean no and unconsciously sabotage his progress.

11

When He's
Not Getting Better

What if you have worked diligently on helping your partner overcome his problem and you see little or no improvement? Things may be going wrong for a number of reasons. Perhaps you are simply being impatient. It usually takes time for a sexual problem to develop, and it takes time for a new way of responding sexually to take its place. Another possibility is that the problem you perceive is not the real problem. A man may appear to have an erection difficulty when he is actually suffering from a desire disorder. A man who is sexually inexperienced may be hiding a paraphilia. A man with extreme premature ejaculation may be covering up an erection problem.

His problem may also go deeper than you think. An extreme case of premature ejaculation can be due to a tremendous amount of sexual guilt, just as certain erection problems can be caused by serious underlying conflicts about women. In some cases these conflicts can be strong enough to prevent resolution of the problem without professional intervention.

There may also be other psychological problems that need to be addressed first. Obsessive-compulsive disorders (OCD) and panic disorders are not uncommon among men with sexual problems. OCD is an insidious problem that makes it almost impossible for the man who has it to focus on pleasurable sexual activity. That is because extraneous and often painful thoughts uncontrollably and pervasively enter his mind. A panic disorder is an extreme anxiety problem that causes the man who has it to obsess about his sexual functioning far more than even the most anxious anticipator.

These disorders are often the primary precipitating cause of a man's sexual dysfunction and need to be treated before a sexual problem can be successfully resolved. Sadly these difficulties are so shameful to the men who have them that they remain largely hidden and undiagnosed. This is particularly true of obsessive-compulsive disorders. Many individuals with this problem believe that they are crazy, so they often keep their fears and problems to themselves. This can lead to a tremendous amount of needless pain and frustration.

For example, Michael was a twenty-six-year-old virgin who was unable to sustain an erection. He had seen three therapists and two physicians before he came to me for treatment. The physicians had told him that there was nothing wrong with him physically, and the therapists all had insisted that extreme performance anxiety was the culprit. But try as he might, the exercises intended to reduce performance anxiety had little positive effect. That is because Michael's problem was not a standard case of performance anxiety at all. When I questioned him about what he was thinking about when he was with a woman, tears sprang to his eyes. "I think about all kinds of things that I do not want to think about. Thoughts just seem to come into my mind and I cannot get rid of them." It did not take long for me to suspect that he was suffering from an obsessive-compulsive disorder. Once Michael's OCD was treated with behavioral and drug therapy, he was able to overcome his problem, and today he has a steady girlfriend.

Your partner may be suffering from OCD if:

- It is extremely difficult for him to focus.
- He cannot clear his mind of invasive thoughts.
- As a child, or an adult, he engaged in any sort of ritualistic behavior.

If you have any reason to believe that the man in your life is suffering with this disorder, suggest that he see a psychologist or psychopharmacologist specializing in OCD as soon as possible. Any major hospital in your vicinity is a good place to begin networking to find such an individual.

Panic disorder is somewhat easier to recognize. There is reason to suspect that a man suffers from panic attacks if:

- He becomes dizzy or faint or has heart palpitations in any high anxiety situation.
- He becomes so unnerved during sex that he feels disoriented and cannot continue.
- He hyperventilates.

Like OCD, panic disorders are treatable. A man who suffers from panic attacks does not necessarily have any deep or serious psychological problems. However, his level of anxiety may be so intense as to preclude working on his sexual problem until his nervousness is reduced to a more manageable level.

BEWARE OF SABOTAGE!

Although an undiagnosed or misdiagnosed problem can certainly prevent you from accomplishing your goals, the most common reason that the program does not succeed is an unconscious resistance to success. Consciously you and your partner may be entirely committed to working through the problem together. Unconsciously one, the other, or both of you may have a stake in not resolving the problem. Either of you may sabotage your progress in an effort to keep the problem alive.

Sabotage comes in all forms. Below are the most common:

- *One or both of you just can't seem to find the time.* This is by far the most common form of resistance to change. In fact, it is astounding that couples who seem to find time for everything else are suddenly at a loss when it comes to putting aside a few hours a week to work on their problem. Barb and Sam, a couple in their early thirties, are a perfect example. Originally they both seemed enthusiastic about working on Sam's premature ejaculation and agreed to set aside a minimum of two hours a week to do it. The first week everything went fine. The second week, however, they had only an hour because the baby had been teething and Barb complained she was exhausted. The third week they did not do the exercises at all, citing a weeklong visit by Sam's parents as their excuse. They felt uncomfortable "working on sex," as Sam put it, when there were parents in close proximity. As I questioned them and we thought about it together, it became obvious to the pair that this was a poor excuse to avoid having to do something that was uncomfortable. Their house was a spacious trilevel, and the guest suite, where Sam's parents were sleeping, was on the lowest level while Sam and Barb's bedroom was on the top.

A similar phenomenon is at work when a couple cannot keep their therapy appointments. It is amazing how couples who have little trouble making their appointments initially can suddenly be on such disparate schedules that it is weeks before they can see me. One couple I was treating for her desire disorder and his inhibited orgasm went through the first four sessions without a hitch. Then, suddenly, the husband, who was in the advertising business, seemed to be available for an appointment only when his wife was busy with an activity involving the children. Finally, since the husband's schedule seemed intractable, I suggested they get additional child care to help cart the kids to and from their activities. This worked for a number of weeks, until the husband's schedule changed again, leaving him time for an appointment only on Friday—a day of the week I do not have office hours!

Unless you are bedridden or in the midst of a life crisis, there is no excuse for not putting aside the necessary time to work on the problem. People make time for what they want to do. Just as you go to work or to the doctor when you need to, you can put aside time to work on your sex life if you really want to. It is a matter of priorities. If you do not have the time, what you or he is saying is that you do not want to make the time.

- *You start a fight, or pick an unpleasant topic of conversation, or bring old grievances to mind when it is time to do the exercises.* This is another very common form of resistance. By creating another problem to focus on, you give yourself what appears to be a legitimate excuse for not working on your sex life. After all, you cannot be therapeutic or sexual when you are angry.
- *You get impatient quickly.* There is very little that can put a man under greater pressure than a partner who complains that overcoming the problem is taking too long. If you do things like heave a heavy sigh when things do not proceed as well as you would like or begin complaining early in the process that you don't know if you can deal with the time it is going to take to solve the problem, the pressure you are putting on your partner will almost guarantee failure.
- *You veer off the program in the name of spontaneity or love.* A lot of people who are unconsciously afraid of resolving their problems try to rush through the process or skip steps along the way. At first you may tell yourself that you do not need to move as slowly as prescribed. This may be true in some cases, but if you are charging ahead and making very little progress, you are engaged in sabotage.

  People who sabotage in this way do so in very creative and insidious ways. For example, a woman whose husband has suffered from long-term premature ejaculation wakes him up in the middle of the night for a "quickie." Or a wife whose husband has been suffering from erection problems attempts intercourse long before he's ready, claiming that she loves him and just needs to feel him inside her.
- *Your words say, "I'll help you," but your actions say, "This is a drag."* As the saying goes, "It's not what you say but what you do." Some men have complained that although their partners follow the steps in the program, they do so with a kind of boredom or indifference that makes the men feel that they are

not really there with them. One man told me that his wife did the manual stop-start exercise with the enthusiasm of dusting a lamp. Another patient told me that as his wife waited for his erection to dissipate before restimulating him, she fell asleep. Yet another said that his wife bartered her participation in the program in exchange for a daily back massage and a new diamond wedding band. The response of a man who meets up with this lack of enthusiasm is likely to be something along the lines of "Don't do me any favors." And though he may very much want to resolve the problem, he may begin to believe that he cannot resolve it with you.

• *You come out with little slips of the tongue that put the heat on.* If there is anything that a man with a sexual problem does not need, it is added pressure. But many women make comments that increase the pressure to perform tenfold. One premature ejaculator, for example, told me that his fiancée had been so happy with his newfound control that she started keeping score of how often she came before he did.

  Dan's experience was even more ego-debilitating. He had suffered on and off from erection difficulties with Robin since the beginning of their relationship. By the time they came for help, their situation had deteriorated to the point that Dan was experiencing such intense performance anxiety that he had not been able to maintain an erection with Robin for four months. After a number of sessions Dan began responding, and a month into treatment he finally achieved penetration and orgasm. He was ecstatic. Robin responded, "Wouldn't it be great to be able to do that twice in a row?" Not surprisingly the next several attempts at intercourse were unsuccessful.

• *You up the ante.* This is an insidious form of sabotage. I have seen women whose partners have erection problems, and who have reported being able to reach orgasm with various forms of stimulation, suddenly proclaiming that their partners' penises are the only way to really satisfy them. There are also women whose partners suffer from PE who begin thrusting wildly during intercourse, now claiming that nothing but a quick in-and-out motion is satisfying to them.

Then, of course, there are men, usually those suffering from inhibited sexual desire, who begin demanding that their partners experience intravaginal orgasm in order for them to be sufficiently turned on. All these new conditions are a way of stopping progress and sabotaging sexual success.

• *New obstacles suddenly appear.* One man, for example, who had been suffering from erection problems and was finally starting to regain functioning, decided that using a condom for contraception was going to prevent him from resolving his problems. It is true that some men do not like condoms, and in some cases the condom can interfere with resolving an erection difficulty. What was striking in this case, however, is that he had already reached penetration with his wife using a condom. In addition, over the years his wife had shown a sensitivity to all forms of birth control. She developed chronic yeast infections with a diaphragm, pelvic inflammatory disease from an IUD, and numerous side effects from the pill. Her husband's new complaint about using a condom and about his wife's negative reaction to it was his unconscious way of resisting treatment.

• *One of you makes yourself less attractive sexually.* If, soon after you start working on the problem, you notice that you are putting on weight or have gotten into wearing a bathrobe that your dog has enjoyed chewing, or that you or your partner stops paying enough attention to physical hygiene, there is little doubt that you are sabotaging any attempt to resolve the problem. The mechanics of actually having to "work on sex" can take enough of the zing out of one's sex life without any added drains.

WHY WOULD YOU OR HE RESIST
GETTING BETTER?

Men and women are often not only unable to see that they are sabotaging their progress but also at a complete loss about why they might be doing so. After all, if there is a problem that can be solved, why would you *not* want to solve it?

The answer is that an individual or a couple may have come to benefit from the presence of the problem in an unconscious way. It is important to understand these gains and work through the resistance that is holding you back from moving forward.

The following are a few of the possible secondary benefits that you or your partner may be deriving from holding on to the problem:

- *You may fear losing your partner if he resolves his problem.* A woman, particularly if she doubts her sexual desirability, may feel very threatened by the prospect of her partner's becoming sexually functional. As one woman in her late forties who had put on a good deal of weight since getting married twenty years before put it, "In a funny way, the fact that he is having trouble with his erections makes me feel safe. I know I am not as attractive as I used to be, and I suppose that deep down I feel that if my husband is uncertain about his potency, he will be less likely to become involved sexually with someone else."

- *You are afraid you will not be able to satisfy your partner sexually.* A woman who has suspected for a long time that her basic lack of sexual interest or responsiveness is a source of disgruntlement for her partner is also likely to experience some secondary gain from keeping him dysfunctional. Responsive men like responsive women. So if you have trouble reaching orgasm or are not that interested in sex, you may be afraid that once he is better, you will not be able to match his level of sexual desire.

- *Focusing on your sexual difficulties can be a distraction from other volatile issues in the relationship.* Sometimes keeping a sexual problem alive is a way of giving a couple something to fight about and focus on, as opposed to dealing with what might *really* be wrong in their relationship. One couple that I had worked with for a period of months, and that had fought about very little else besides the husband's premature ejaculation problem, began arguing about having children as soon as his ejaculatory control began to improve. The fact that he wanted children and she did not had been an unresolved sore spot in their relationship since they had married five years before. Their lack of agreement on this issue was potentially devastating to the relationship. Rather than deal with the real problem, the wife started refusing to work on the exercises that were accounting for her husband's progress, under the ruse that she was now enjoying sex less because of the effort that she had to put into it. Not surprisingly, when her husband's PE started worsening again, she began demeaning him for having the problem to begin with.

- *You don't want to solve the problem because it gives an otherwise empty relationship a point of focus.* In relationships in which two people either have never been close or have grown apart, a problem can be the last thread holding them together. Although having a sexual problem undoubtedly creates tension, fighting about it provides an area of joint interest when there is no other common ground. If this is your situation, you may fear that if the problem is solved, there will be nothing to talk about at all.

- *Harping on his problem can be a distraction from dealing with* your *sexual problems.* In the same way that a sexual problem can distract a couple from other issues in their relationship, a man's sexual problem can take the heat off his partner if she has a sexual dysfunction. Many men are very protective of their partners, and I have been struck by how often a man would prefer to take the hit for being sexually dysfunctional than push his partner to deal with her problem.

- *His problem complements a hidden lack of desire on your part.* Over the years I have discovered that a lot of women for various reasons have lost interest in sex. Instinctively they know, however, that to present one's self as not desiring sex and being sexually undesirable could lead to infidelity on the part of one's mate. The sexual problem that the partner of such a woman has feeds right into her lack of desire, giving her a legitimate excuse for not wanting to have sex.

The same is true for a woman who has lost interest not in sex but only in her long-term partner. If she is engaged in the heat of an extramarital liaison, the development of a partner's sexual problem is likely to be met with a sigh of relief. As one fifty-six-year-old grandmother who had been involved with a forty-three-year-old man for two years put it, "When my husband, who is sixty-five, started having trouble with his erections, it gave me a real excuse not to be interested anymore. Of course," she added, "he thought I had been sexually washed up for years anyway."

- *His problem is a cover-up for his loss of attraction.* Of course, loss of interest can work both ways. A man who has lost interest in his wife yet is not prepared to look for sex outside the marriage may opt to retain his sexual difficulty. Unconsciously it is easier for him to have a sexual problem than to deal with the lack of desire for his spouse.

- *Keeping your partner sexually dysfunctional may be your way of gaining power in your relationship.* Regina is a case in point. I will never forget the day that she strutted into my office with her multimillionaire husband and said flat-out, "Here. You fix him." Regina complained that she had lived with her husband's premature ejaculation for twenty years and was tired of what she viewed as his lack of sexual consideration. I spent a number of sessions with her husband, Paul, going over the various exercises that would help him gain better control. We also spent a good deal of time talking about the various ways a man could pleasure a woman. Paul finally got up the courage to try out some of his newly learned skills with Regina. But it was to no avail. "Well, he lasts longer that he used to," Regina said sarcastically the next time the three of us met. "But I can't stand the way that he kisses. He sticks his tongue down my throat. He slobbers all over me." When I suggested that Regina show Paul how she liked to be kissed, she was completely resistant to the idea. "I told you," she said. "*You* fix him."

After months of fighting the idea, Regina finally agreed to have a private session with me. What emerged was a woman who felt completely powerless in her marriage. Although she lived in a ten-thousand-square-foot mansion and her husband made millions, she told me that he controlled access to the money and that she was required to ask him each week for her "allowance." It became obvious that Regina's desire to keep Paul sexually inept was, in her mind, the only way that she could have any control in the relationship.

- *One of you is nervous about failing.* Even when the motivation to solve the problem is high, one or the other party may hear a little voice in his or her head that says, "What if this doesn't work?" The fear, of course, is that if the problem is not resolved, the relationship will end. Although not working on the problem prevents you from ever having to deal with this potential threat, it also obliterates the possibility that things might get better.

If you suspect that one of you is experiencing any of the problems I've just described, then it is detrimental to continue working on it without professional intervention. Unconsciously sabotaging the progress of a man with a sexual problem is worse than doing nothing at all because you are undermining a person whose confidence is already shaken.

Since your man's sexual problem is your problem too, if you're in a relationship with him, seeking help together is the best strategy. The American Association of Sex Educators, Counselors, and Therapists is headquartered in Chicago and will provide you with a list of qualified professionals in your geographic area.

If your partner refuses to go with you, it's a good idea for you to speak to a therapist on your own. You may gain some insight into whether you are contributing to the problem and, if so, what steps you might take to turn things around. At the very least you may be able to figure out if you are willing to live with the status quo.

SEX AFTER PROBLEMS

Although it may take a little time, chances are that your partner will eventually commit to resolving his sexual problem. Often, this is less a reflection of a man's desire to save his relationship than it is on his ego. I have worked with scores of men who were the ones who initiated therapy. Of course, their partners were not thrilled about the presence of a sexual difficulty and were happy to be taking steps to alleviate it. But they were generally less disturbed about the problem than the man himself was.

Regardless of who takes the first step toward better sexual functioning, life after working through a sexual problem holds many rewards.

Better Sex

This may seem obvious. After all, problem-free sex has to be better than when there is something wrong or the fear of a problem to contend with. But sex improves in many other unanticipated ways as well.

Many couples begin experiencing a freedom of sexual expression that they never had before. Working on a sexual problem with a partner requires direct and open communication and takes a lot of the hush-hush out of sex. Sharing sexual wants and needs during lovemaking becomes easier and less embarrassing. Many couples that I have worked with also develop a more experimental attitude toward sex.

"The fact that Arthur can last a lot longer now is only one of the benefits of having dealt with his premature ejaculation problem," one woman who had initially been quite disturbed about her husband's lack of control and was now delighted about his progress told me at our final session. "I feel a lot less shy than I used to when it comes to sex. I suddenly find myself asking Arthur to touch me in a certain way or in a certain place right at the moment that I want him to. Arthur and I both noticed that I am also making a lot more noise when I come. I suppose that having had to talk about all this stuff in order to work on Arthur's PE has made me less embarrassed about sex in a lot of ways."

Many people also find that their lovemaking becomes more varied and exciting. "We both used to think that intercourse was the equivalent of having sex," said Mike, whose erection problems were resolved after his wife, Jane, overcame her ignorance about a man's need for genital stimulation. "I'm not saying that intercourse isn't great, but it isn't the goal. The result is that our sex life has become a lot more spontaneous and less predictable. Sometimes we come with petting, sometimes we bring each other to orgasm orally, and sometimes we screw. It's a lot more fun because we are never sure when we start where we are going to end up."

A More Intimate Relationship

Another advantage of working on a sexual problem to a successful outcome is that a relationship often becomes closer emotionally.

Communication generally becomes better, for one thing. "Working on Ron's sexual problem has really taught us how to talk to each other," said Jackie, after six months of therapy geared toward alleviating her husband's combined difficulties with erections and premature ejaculation. "Ron used to keep a lot of things to himself. But you can't do that and solve a sexual problem. He's much more open now and is also a much better listener." Ron concurred. "If you can talk about the gory details of your sex life—'play with my balls, not so hard, faster, slower, stop, start'—then nothing's taboo."

The process of resolving a sexual problem also provides a strong foundation for dealing with other problems. There are many components that are essential to overturning a sexual problem: patience, commitment, an ability to listen, suspending judgment, a sense of humor. The process of working together on a sexual problem requires that you develop and fine tune these skills. So when you are done solving a sexual problem, you have a tool box that you can carry with you and use while working on other aspects of your relationship.

Finally, the power of having survived and conquered a problem together is very bonding. It takes a lot of commitment for a woman to stick things out through the rough spots, and a lot of men feel a greater commitment to their partners as a result.

For Calvin, a man with an orgasm problem, his partner's acceptance of his problem and cooperation in solving it was what clinched his decision to marry her. "I never doubted whether I loved Kristie, but when I first met her I did have some questions about her emotional maturity. She had three different jobs in three years. I suppose I wondered if she had trouble sticking things out, and that concerned me." Kristie's dedication and hard work over many months to help Calvin resulted in Calvin's ability to have orgasm intravaginally for the first time in his life, and convinced him that Kristie did have more than ample stick-to-itiveness. They have been married now for two years, during which time Kristie started a successful home day-care center.

A More Sensitive Man

Although I would never wish having a sexual problem on any male, there is little doubt that there is something different and special about a man who has overcome such a problem.

My own observations, as well as those of their partners, lead me to believe that men who deal with their sexual problems in a straight-forward way become stronger yet gentler men. The simple admission that he has a problem confronts a man with his own vulnerability. Letting me or another woman in on the problem and how he feels about it forces him to let down his guard. Taking the risk of sharing his innermost feelings and insecurities so that he can work through the problem gives him first-hand experience with what it is like to be truly intimate.

It's a hard way to learn a lesson, but the benefit is often a man's feeling that he does not have to be macho to be masculine. He can be vulnerable and still have a woman's respect. He can show his feelings and not be emasculated. All told, the man who has the courage to tackle a sexual problem becomes a man who needs to prove less and who can love more.

Of course, there are some men who seem to revert to the old bravado as soon as the problem goes away. "In a strange sense, Sam and I were closer when we were dealing with his erection problem than ever before," one woman confessed. "He's a powerful man in business, very much used to being in control of things. But having trouble getting hard seemed to humble him. It gave him a softer edge . . . no pun intended." Things changed after Sam's erection problem was solved. "He seemed to go back to the way he was before. It was almost as if everything we had gone through dealing with the problem—the tears, the talking, the emotional closeness—was forgotten. It's almost like he had never had a problem at all."

I have had similar experiences. I always request that a patient call me two to four months after finishing therapy just to let me know how things are going. While most men readily comply, there are some who not only do not call, but refuse to return my calls when I take the initiative. Others call, but are curt, emotionless, and at face value, downright unappreciative.

Over the years, however, I have learned to understand that it is not that they are ungrateful. They simply want to forget. Having a sexual problem can be such a blow to the ego that once resolved, a man may want to wipe any trace or recollection of it from memory. He does not want to remember what feeling frightened and vulnerable was like. He does not want to think about having exposed himself emotionally to me. But somewhere, of course, I know he knows. And he knows that I know, and that he really doesn't have to worry.

His secrets are safe with me.

Index

ABOUT THE AUTHOR

Eva Margolies, M.A., C.S.T., is the director of the Center for Sexual Recovery in New York City. She is one of the nation's most prominent sex therapists and is certified by the American Association of Sex Educators, Counselors, and Therapists. Author of five books on men, women, and sexuality, including *Sensual Pleasure* and *The Samson and Delilah Complex*, she has been featured in *People Magazine* and has appeared as an expert on *20/20*, *The Today Show*, *Oprah*, and CNBC.